SHERLOCK AND I

A Memoir of Medical Mysteries

in a Rural U.S. Practice

By Frederick Kassis, M.D.

D1534231

Sherlock and I:

A Memoir of Medical Mysteries in a Rural U.S. Practice

By Frederick Kassis, M.D.

DEDICATION

I practiced rural medicine for almost forty years. During that time I had the distinct pleasure of caring for people with varied conditions, and I learned about the strength of the human soul. My patients taught me much about courage in the way they bore their often terrible illnesses. They also taught me the meaning of compassion, as I watched them care for their ill family members. During those years, I saw my patients through many crises – emotional and medical. I had to be there to help them into the next life, by allowing them to die with dignity. That was the most difficult part of my job, since so many of these people had become my friends – people who I truly looked forward to seeing in the office. Now that I have retired, I miss them greatly. I dedicate this book to all of them.

I need also to dedicate this book to Peggy Hansen, a brilliant and talented nurse consultant, without whose encouragement I would have never began such a project. Unfortunately Peggy lost her battle with lung cancer on January 14, 2017, thus depriving the world of her marvelous intelligence, expertise in almost every aspect of nursing care, her wonderful wit, and her enthusiasm for life in general. She is greatly missed by all who knew her.

Frederick J Kassis, MD

CHAPTER 1

THE BEGINNINGS

I entered medical school in 1966 thinking I wanted to be a plastic surgeon; however, my rotation through surgery as a third-year medical student had made me realize that I truly hated surgery. I found that I did not have the patience to stand for hours doing very tedious work. But, when I got to my internal medicine rotation I knew that I had found my calling. These doctors were, indeed, detectives: they sorted through a myriad of clues contained in the patient's history and laboratory data, examined the patient, and, by so doing, developed a plausible list of diagnoses together with both an investigative and a treatment plan. I was hooked. For years I had read *The Great Adventures of Sherlock Holmes*, by Sir Arthur Conan Doyle; now I had found a segment of medical science that would allow me to emulate my hero. What could be better?

During my fourth year of medical school at Loyola-Stritch Medical School, I applied for and was accepted to a hematology clerkship At UC Davis Medical Center in Sacramento, California. During that clerkship, I managed to read *Wintrobe's Clinical Hematology* tome from cover to cover – No small feat. However, although I learned so much during that rotation, I found out that, as a hematologist, I would also have to do cancer therapy, since oncology was a part of that specialty. There was no way that my psyche could handle that.

But the better result of that rotation was that the faculty at UC Davis decided that they really liked me, and offered me a residency in internal medicine, which I readily accepted.

So by the end of June, 1975, I had completed my three-year residency training in internal medicine. Those years were marked by chronic sleep deprivation, as we were often "on call" for forty-eight to seventy-two hours at a time. However, the training was excellent; and, after passing my board exam, I felt like I was ready to enter the world of private practice. Davis had offered me a fellowship in cardiology. I, however, was interested in the whole of internal medicine, and could not see myself limited to just one aspect of that discipline, when there were a myriad of other diagnoses that needed to be considered in the management of a patient's health.

So, having declined that, I looked for a place to practice. I had always geared my approach to the study of medicine toward practice in a rural setting. I was attracted to practice in a small town because I thought that, with my additional medical knowledge, I could make a significant difference to the people living there, who so often struggled to recruit and retain physicians. As an internist, I knew that I could bring a special expertise to such a community, which so often had only family practice physicians delivering their medical care. I knew that I would not have subspecialists at my beck and call to bail me out of difficult problems. I had studied feverishly during my training, so that I would feel secure in my approach to medical care. I would need to rely heavily on my physical examination skills in that setting, since I would lack many of the sophisticated studies available to me at the university. My search finally landed me and my wife and two small boys in a small town in southern Idaho known as Rupert, with a population of slightly over five thousand. The town is located on the northern side of the Snake River, as it wends its way through the southern part of the state. Irrigation canals crisscross the farmlands that surround the town, and a sugar-beet processing plant two miles from the town added economic stability to the area. Across the river lays the slightly larger town of Burley, with its population of ten thousand, so the overall drawing area -- considering all of the adjacent farms -- was thirty thousand people.

There was no internal medicine physician in the area. Eventually, my profession would take me to another small town in west Texas named Sweetwater, where I would practice during the last fifteen years of my career; however, I began my professional journey in the high desert area where Rupert is located.

Rupert is the county seat of Minidoka County. Minidoka Memorial Hospital in Rupert recruited me to the town, and offered me a startup stipend until I could make enough money to be on my own. A family physician had recently left the area, and I was able to occupy his office. However, although I felt pretty secure in my medical knowledge, I quickly realized that I knew nothing at all about the business of running a medical practice. Somehow, my medical school and residency training had taught me nothing about those aspects of medicine. Fortunately, the office manager from the previous practice agreed to work for me, and she began to show me the ropes. I had so many questions, for example, "What is the 'franchise tax thing?" I had no clue about how much it cost to run a medical practice in those days. I had no concept of how to bill for my services. I ended up calling one of the internists in Twin Falls, which was about forty miles from me, to ask him how he charged for his time and services. Fortunately, he was nice enough to give me that information, so that now I probably wasn't going to starve. At times, though, I felt like I was treading water in the vast expanses of the ocean of business.

I remember thinking to myself that, now that I had left the university setting, I probably would not see too many interesting problems any more. I found out during the first week of my practice how wrong I was about this. Indeed, my many years of rural practice would offer me innumerable medical challenges, many of which would test my abilities as a physician far more than they had ever been tested during my training years. They were years filled with nonstop learning, as I continued to read medical journals avidly to expand my medical knowledge in order to care for the numerous problems that I had not yet encountered during my training years; and, indeed there were many of those... The hospital that recruited me was a small, twenty-five bed facility that provided both routine radiology and laboratory services. However, there was no CT scanner on the premises. The other hospital located across the river in Burley, was double the size; yet it also lacked a CT scanner. The nearest hospital of any size was located forty miles away in Twin Falls; however it lacked an invasive cardiologist. The nearest neurosurgeon resided in Pocatello – seventy-five miles away. Cardiology expertise was to be found in Boise, a two-and-one-half hour drive from us. I discovered – much to my dismay – that there was no air-transport company servicing the region, so that all transfers would have to be done by ground ambulance... It seemed, indeed, that Fate had definitely granted my wish; this was to be truly a practice of "rural medicine."

The good news was that there were two general surgeons who covered the two hospitals – Leo Brown, who lived in Rupert, and Hayden Ellingham, who practiced in Burley. Both of them had been in the service, and had served in the Vietnam conflict. I was to discover later that these two men were really "pro's," who were comfortable performing both routine surgical procedures and caring, as well, for patients suffering major trauma. In addition, they got along well, and often operated together if the occasion called for it. For the rest of my medical career I would always compare my surgical consultants to these two extremely skilled surgeons!

The hospital administrator informed me, after I had arrived, that I would have to take "ER call," as part of my being credentialed at the hospital. At that time, there were no permanent emergency physicians who covered the emergency room. The real surprise was that he expected me to see children as well as adults who presented there. Now, I had had a month of pediatric training during my residency, but had not seen any children since my first year of that training. I paled with fear at the thought of caring for a sick child. I tried my best to get out of doing that; however, the administrator would not relent. There were four other family physicians in the community, who admitted patients to the hospital and who shared the ER coverage duties. So, at least, I would not be doing this every night.

I realized that I had to update my knowledge of pediatrics very quickly, so I ordered a manual of emergency pediatric management, and, when it arrived, I devoured it over a period of a week. By then, I felt that I could at least keep a child from dying in the ER until I could get them to the pediatrician in Twin Falls. This knowledge would come in handy sooner than I expected. This manual would later help me to save a young child's live at a time when I thought, for certain, that he was a goner…

I was in my office on Monday, getting things organized so that I could open my door for business the next day, when the action suddenly began for me. The phone rang; it was Richard Johnson the hospital radiologist calling to ask if I could come over immediately to help him with a patient who had gone into shock after receiving a dye that would image his kidneys. He told me that the patient was still on the x-ray table and that he had a blood pressure of 50/0. I replied that I would be right over, but that he should quickly move the patient to the ER, where I could treat him more easily. I then hurried over to the emergency room to see what was going on.

CHAPTER 2

A MATTER OF SHOCK

A naphylaxis. Even the word itself sounds ominous – as, indeed, is the condition. Imagine that you have a bucket that is filled with water up to the top. Now imagine that the size of that bucket suddenly doubles. Your now have a half-full bucket. That is exactly what happens when a patient has an anaphylactic attack. Suddenly, in response to an antigen stimulus, all of the patient's blood vessels suddenly lose the diameter that they maintained before the stimulus came along, and they expand. Therefore, the blood that is contained in those vessels now is contained in a "bigger bucket," and the patient's blood pressure – which used to be normal at 120/70 -- now drops to extremely low levels, or may even become unobtainable. The stimulus that triggered this lethal string of events might be a bee sting, peanut products, or, as in this case, the contrast material that is injected in order to visualize different organs such as the brain and the kidneys. The end result of this rapidly developing process is that the heart cannot develop enough pressure to propel the blood to the organs that need it – the brain, heart, intestines, and extremities -- all of which cannot survive without the oxygen- carrying blood. The patient is now in a "shock" state, in which his tissues are suddenly deprived of their oxygen. The brain begins to falter, and the patient becomes confused. The heart struggles to respond to this problem by increasing its rate, thereby trying to fill up the blood vessel tree. The kidneys begin to fail, and stop making any urine. The extremities, deprived of their blood supply, become cool, blue, and mottled. All systems begin to fail – and this process occurs over a matter of a few minutes. Ultimately the heart no longer adequately compensate for this self-sustaining lethal process, since it, too, depends on a head of pressure in the blood vessels that bring blood to its surface; it finally ceases to contract. At this point, the patient is now gone. When it happens in front of you, it is very dramatic; and, if you are a physician observing all of this, your anal sphincter begins to pucker. I had treated anaphylaxis many times during my residency, so this problem was certainly not new to me. However, each time a physician is faced with this horrible catastrophe, he hopes and prays that the medications and fluids that are about to be administered to reverse the problem will actually work. Most of the time, they do. However, as I was to discover a couple of years later, there are rare occasions when none of your efforts to change the patient's downhill course will prevail, and he or she dies.

When I arrived in the ER, I found the local photographer John Snelling lying on a gurney. John had lived in Rupert all of his life. He had become interested in photography in high school, and, over time, had become the best photographer in town, with most families employing him to shoot their family portraits. I had met him, along with his family about a week before at a local café. He was about five feet nine inches tall, balding, and covered the entire gurney. Sweat poured from every pore of his face and torso. His blue eyes were widely opened; he was agitated, and kept changing his position on the gurney. ER nurses surrounded the man on the gurney, each one looking very worried. One of them was checking his IV to be sure that it was working. Another nurse was anxiously looking at the monitor, which kept flashing John's abnormal vital signs. A respiratory therapist was placing an oxygen mask over his face. The blood pressure measured 60/0 – truly defining the "shock state" in which he was currently existing. His body was trying with all of its might to maintain life in him. Because his brain was lacking its normal oxygen supply, he was somewhat confused, and answered my questions with monosyllabic responses. "Have you ever had any allergies to anything before?" I asked. He mumbled. "No." I further questioned him and learned that he had no history of heart problems, blood pressure issues, or diabetes. Although it certainly looked like John was in the throes of an anaphylactic attack, I had to consider other diagnoses as well. Had he suffered a heart attack, which had killed heart muscle to the point that it could not contract effectively? Had he been born with an abnormal heart valve, which had worsened to the point where it was no longer allowing blood to flow forward? Was a pulmonary embolus to blame, where blood clots travel to the lungs and act as a dam, preventing blood from flowing to through the lungs? Was there any evidence of overwhelming infection, which could also dilate his blood vessels, as does the anaphylactic cascade.

John did not have risk factors that would support the embolus theory – he had not been traveling on a plane, nor had he been lying in a bed in the hospital for a while; so blood clots probably had not formed in his legs. He had no family history of blood clots.

His wife now arrived in the emergency room. A woman of about five feet two inches, with brown eyes and hair, she was dressed in a white blouse tucked into a light brown pair of slacks. She was obviously upset, but still calm enough to help me out with John's medical history. She was able to tell me that he did not have risk factors for a heart attack: high blood pressure, elevated cholesterol, or diabetes. Additionally, she informed me that her husband had seen his doctor two days before this episode, complaining of abdominal pain, and was diagnosed as having a kidney stone – hence the reason for the test that he had today. He had not complained about having chills, which would suggest an infection.

I now began my examination, while, at the same time ordering an EKG, chest x-ray, and blood work to look for evidence of a heart attack as well as to evaluate his kidney function, electrolytes (sodium and potassium levels), and his complete blood count. The latter could give me a clue as to whether or not infection may be present. Starting at his feet and legs, I found very cool and mottled skin, and his pulses in the groin were not palpable. His abdomen was soft, and I did not elicit any winces from him when I pushed on it. I heard some wheezes in his chest, but he was having not pain in the chest when he took a breath – again suggesting that he had not suffered a pulmonary embolus. He could move his arms and legs well; so that, although he was a little mentally slow at this time, this suggested that he had not suffered a stroke. Lastly, I began a careful auscultation of his heart. This organ was pumping regularly, and the familiar "lub-dub" sound was clearly present. I heard no "swooshing" sound that would tell me that he had a valve problem. However, his blood pressure was 60/0, and his heart rate was 118. Fortunately for him, his oxygen level was still in the low normal range of 90 percent.

An anaphylactic attack is truly one of those "medical emergencies" that are written about in the medical literature. It strikes terror in the hearts of both the patient and the physician. In treating this problem, I had to accomplish two objectives. First of all, I had to fill up his "bucket." Secondly, I had to administer medications that would not only help to reverse the deadly process, but also help sustain his blood pressure. To accomplish the first goal, I ordered the staff to give John infusions of two bottles of saline solution. That would begin to fill up his overly-dilated vascular system, and, by so-doing, begin to raise his blood pressure. I now had to try to reverse the deadly process.

I swiftly ordered the staff to give John epinephrine in order to squeeze his blood vessels, thereby helping to raise his blood pressure as well as to help his heart pump more strongly. Along with these measures I had to administer additional medications that would help to reverse the deadly process in which John was involved. Epinephrine is always the first-line drug; however, I also had to add an antihistamine such as Benadryl, which would act immediately to block receptors involved in the reaction. Lastly I needed to administer a hydrocortisone type medication which would gradually reverse the effects that the dye was having on the receptors in his blood vessels. I ordered the nurse to administer that drug along with the others and to place a catheter into his bladder in order to monitor his urine output. (It would actually be a number of hours yet before the steroid medication would begin to take full effect, and John would receive doses every six hours in order to prevent any relapse of the anaphylaxis.) It was the epinephrine, along with the fluids and the Benadryl that I was hoping would work their magic immediately, and begin to get John out of trouble.

By now I had received some results from his early studies. His "cardiac enzyme" blood test revealed no evidence for heart damage. I saw no signs of fluid or infection in his lung on reviewing his chest x-ray, and I noticed that his white blood cell count was only minimally above normal at 11,100 – suggesting that infection was unlikely.

So, by this time I was pretty secure with my diagnosis: John was suffering from an anaphylactic reaction to the intravenous contrast, which had been given to him in order to outline his kidneys and their drainage system. I had administered all of the appropriate fluids and medications in order to stabilize him; it was now just a waiting game to see if these measures were going to work. Now it was our turn to sweat.

Most of the time the medications do their job, and the patient improves; however, this improvement – if it occurs – takes time. And so we waited, and waited – and waited longer.

Gradually John's blood pressure slowly began to climb – 70/20; 82/30; 90/34, until finally, after about thirty-five minutes, he reached 102/58. With this improvement, John became more mentally alert, and his profuse sweating began to resolve. His kidneys even started to make some urine, which fact – along with the other changes that he was demonstrating – told us that we had begun to get decent control of his emergent condition. We had won this particular battle.

John had stabilized for now, but the hydrocortisone-related medication Solu-medrol would not really be at its peak activity for at least another six to eight hours; this is the medication that finally serves to reverse the process and stabilize the patient in this situation. Therefore, I admitted John to the ICU where he could be monitored closely and continue to receive the intravenous Solu-Medrol along with further fluids and Benadryl. I also had to take measures to prevent this catastrophe from happening to him in the future.

By the next morning, John's vital signs were stable, and he was alert and oriented. His lab workup was normal – no evidence for heart damage. Overnight he had passed his kidney stone; so that the precipitating issue was now resolved. After he ate a good breakfast, I discharged him. However, I continued him on the cortisone-type medication for another five days to prevent any relapse. At his subsequent visit with me a week later, I was looking at a healthy man. I made sure that both his office and hospital charts reflected that he was "allergic to contrast," so that he would not have to undergo this emergency condition again. I also asked him get an application from one of the local pharmacies for a wrist band that would indicate that he was "allergic to contrast." I referred him to the urologist, who would evaluate John concerning the kidney stone.

John experienced a disorder that brings people to the hospital very frequently, since the reaction may be triggered by almost any substance foreign to the human   body to which that person's body has been previously exposed – for example, insect bites, medications, bee stings, and foods such as products derived from peanuts. The problem with this disorder lies in how quickly the patient can go from being perfectly healthy to approaching death within a matter of minutes. Immunologists discovered the mechanisms by which the triggering antigens bind with the antibodies within the patient and trigger the release of chemicals from white blood cells many years ago. However, once these chemicals are released, the body's reaction to them occurs so quickly that up to 1 percent may die from this disorder, even in a metropolitan center. Most family physicians do not have to deal with this condition; therefore, they are often not familiar with the treatment methods. Since some of these patients need to be managed on a ventilator if their respiration fails; thus, the patient living in a rural environment is at a higher risk of dying from this acute attack on his or her cardiovascular system. People die with anaphylaxis because they remain in shock and because their lungs often fill with fill with fluid, preventing those lungs from obtaining the oxygen necessary to survive. The ability to deal with this kind of emergency is one of the areas of expertise that, as an internist, I bring to patients living in a rural setting

John Snelling had suffered a catastrophic medical emergency. His acute condition is analogous to a four-alarm fire. The conflagration affects the entire building, and is easily seen by all persons, both near and far. The firemen realize that they will have to do multiple things all at one time in order to contain the blaze; there is no mystery.

Another medical example of this sort of presentation is a patient who presents to the emergency room with a heart attack. That person begins to have chest pain, which – within four to six minutes – becomes quite intense. Besides feeling a distinct heaviness in his or her chest, the patient may commonly experience shortness of breath, nausea, and fairly profuse sweating as well. This conflagration is clearly visible. The confluence of symptoms in this particular patient clearly points to a problem involving that person's heart and/or lungs.

When that patient arrives in the emergency room, the doctor will ask questions about the onset of the pain, radiation of the pain, and about the associated symptoms mentioned above. He or she will ask about risk factors for heart disease – a family history of events, smoking history, blood pressure history, diabetes history, and any history of high cholesterol. The physician will also order an EKG, chest x-ray and laboratory studies looking at that patient's blood count, liver and kidney function, and search for enzymes in the blood that are released from the heart when it is damaged. If the EKG shows evidence for a heart attack and/or the heart enzymes in the blood are elevated, then this patient has a heart attack – a four-alarm fire that presented in a straightforward manner. A disease process – like the anaphylaxis episode presented above – that may rapidly kill the patient who suffers it. The ER physician, along with consultants, must now attack this fire with multiple medications and, perhaps, even interventions such coronary artery stenting or bypass in order to gain control of the disease – the fire -- if you will.

However, there are a myriad of other diseases that do not announce their presence in such a dramatic a manner. There are no fire trucks involved in the treatment of these diseases. That is because these disorders, at first, do not manifest as a blaze. Rather, many of them begin merely as a tiny ember, located deeply inside the body of a patient. This ember, which actually may begin in multiple sites at once, or affect different organs at different times, may smolder for days, weeks, months, or even years before they finally begin to expand their flames to the point where the patient begins to have symptoms. The diseases might involve just one organ, or they may attack many organs at once or in sequence as their flames expand.

The disorders commonly give up to the attending physician the clues to their existence very grudgingly, and often over time; therefore the attending physician (and maybe even his consultants) will frequently have much difficulty arriving at a correct diagnosis, and correct treatment might be significantly delayed – often for years. As we say in medicine, the physician must always maintain a "high index of suspicion" about the possible presence of these disorders in order that he or she might make the correct diagnosis and initiate the proper treatment. But saying that is easy; doing it is a significantly harder task…

I have practiced internal medicine for forty years. I spent thirteen years in Idaho, but then a divorce sent me to Texas in search of a steady paycheck. After a stint of twelve years at the Austin Regional Clinic in Austin, Texas, I finished the last fifteen years of my medical practice at a rural health clinic located in the west Texas town of Sweetwater, Texas. I was finally back to the rural environment that I loved. There I worked with a great group of six physicians, who were clearly dedicated to doing the best job that they could for their patients. As the only internist in the community,

I became their consultant on cases that were giving them trouble. It was here, in Sweetwater, Texas, that I diagnosed many of these "smoldering" diseases that had decided to affect some very sweet, wonderful, and courageous patients. Many of these disorders are considered somewhat rare, statistically speaking. However, I always used to remind the medical students who were with me as well as the patients themselves, "statistics do not apply to the individual patient."

CHAPTER 3

THE FLUTTERING HEART

E ddie Baker was around fifty years old when I first met him. He was well built, about five feet eight inches tall, with dark brown eyes and still sporting all of his hair. He worked a one of the local banks, and was within eight years of retiring from his post there. He exercised fairly regularly, and so appeared to be in better shape than many of the patients who appeared in my examination rooms.

Eddie had developed hypertension about four years ago, and had been seeing one of the local family physicians for treatment of that problem. She had been able to control his blood pressure fairly easily up until about eight months ago, when it began to run significantly higher than usual. She had added a second drug to his regimen; however, his numbers were remaining in the 150/96 range – well above the goal of at least 140/90. Because of this fact, Eddie had decided to visit me, the local internist, to discuss the problem of his hypertension.

I sat down and listened to his story. Except for his blood pressure problem, he seemed to be in good health. He ate a healthy diet and, as mentioned above, participated in regular exercise – usually bike riding with his wife. I asked him further questions concerning his problem; he had no history of kidney disease, which could cause his hypertension. In addition, he was not having any symptoms related to his elevated blood pressure – headaches, shortness of breath, chest pain, swelling in his legs, or heart palpitations. I went over his salt intake (increased salt intake tends to increase blood pressure). Eddie assured me that he was not indulging in eating French fries, potato chips, Fritos, dill pickles, or other high sodium foods. However, he did tend to add salt to his food at the table. His family doctor had prescribed Hydrochlorothiazide, which is known as a "water pill" because it acts on the kidneys to remove extra salt and water from the body, thereby lowering blood pressure. To this she had added Lisinopril (an angiotensin converting-enzyme inhibitor), which has relatively few side effects – the most common of which is a dry, hacking cough). The medication can also affect kidney function and potassium levels in the blood; so she had been monitoring blood tests periodically. Surely, she was practicing good medicine, yet Eddie's blood pressure had not responded to these medication changes.

I now proceeded to examine Mr. Baker. His blood pressure was 148/96 in both arms, while his heart and lungs were completely normal. Upon listening to his flanks and abdomen with my stethoscope, I heard no sounds that would indicate a diminished blood flow to either kidney. His general exam did not suggest any hormonal imbalance. The blood pressure in each arm was identical, and the pulses in his legs indicated excellent blood flow. I did an EKG, which was also normal.

So far, it seemed that Eddie had "essential hypertension," a disorder that afflicts millions of people in the US and elsewhere. It is known as the "silent killer," because a patient's blood pressure might be quite high for a number of years, while he or she has no symptoms. However, untreated hypertension ultimately will lead to those patients having a stroke, heart attack, or other symptoms related to blood vessel damage. Ninety-seven out of one hundred patients who develop hypertension do so for mechanisms that are not fully understood, and are labeled as having "essential hypertension." About three patients out of that one hundred will have an underlying cause for their pressure elevation, which may involve a diminished blood supply to one or more kidneys, chronic kidney disease, or an abnormal release of various hormones from the adrenal gland – which sits like a cap on the top of each kidney.

At the end of his first visit with me, I advised Mr. Baker to cut back further on his salt intake, and I ordered laboratory tests to check his blood count, liver and kidney function, sodium and potassium levels, thyroid levels, cholesterol studies, and a urinalysis. I asked him to return in six weeks for follow up.

At his next visit his blood pressure was now 138/82 – a distinct improvement over before. Eddie was no longer adding salt to his food, and was carefully avoiding the culprits that could increase his blood pressure. His lab work done after his previous visit had returned as normal. At that point, we decided to leave his medications the same, and he would monitor his blood pressure at home, with a follow up visit in six months. I would have liked to see his pressure a little lower; however he was now in the normal range, so I did not add any further medications at this point. In the late seventies all of the insurance companies had published their actuarial data on death and hypertension, which indicated that there was a straight-line relationship; the higher a patient's blood pressure was, the more likely that he or she would die of complications of the disease... There was no cut-off line, below which one was safe and above which one was likely to suffer one of the events mentioned. Therefore, over my years in practice, I always attempted to get my patients' blood pressure levels down around 120/60-70 – if I could do that without giving the patient intolerable side effects. I decided that, if his pressure were not lower at the next visit, then I would adjust his medications further.

Eddie returned in six months as scheduled. He brought with him his blood pressure readings so that I could review them. Most of the readings were in the normal range; but periodically he would have days when his numbers would reach 158/94 and even 168/96. He assured me that he was watching his salt intake, and that he had not developed any new symptoms. His exam that day was once again normal, and I ordered lab tests, which were normal.

We reviewed our options. There was room to increase the angiotensin receptor inhibitor, which should not increase his side effects significantly; so I doubled his dose, and we agreed to meet again in six weeks. I arranged to check his labs in two weeks to be certain that the increase did not affect his kidneys or potassium levels.

Six weeks went by, and Eddie returned for his follow-up visit. Once again he brought his readings with him, which were in the 134/74 range; although he still had a few days when the pressure would hit 156/98. He also had developed a couple of new symptoms: he had noticed some brief episodes of sweating, occurring even at rest, along with some occasional heart palpitations. The sweating episodes might occur once a week or as often as two to three times a day. The palpitations seemed to follow the same pattern. Some of these feelings of palpitations seemed to him just to be an extra heartbeat or two, while at other times he would sense a "run" of extra heartbeats lasting ten to fifteen seconds. At no time did he feel lightheaded or develop chest pain. The sweating episodes might occur in isolation; but sometimes they would happen along with the palpitations. Exercise had no effect on either of his symptoms.

In the office that day his blood pressure was 128/72; once again his exam remained normal. I repeated his EKG and his lab work that day, both of which demonstrated no changes from before. There were no extra heartbeats noted on the EKG. I asked him if I would be able tell when he was having his sweating episodes, and his response was "yes." He even volunteered at this point that sometimes, right before the sweating episodes, he would become pale – something that his wife had even noticed.

And so, at this time, as Sherlock might say, "the plot thickens." I sensed that there was an ember that has been smoldering in this man for a while, and which was now showing signs of increasing in size, as manifested by the additional symptoms that Eddie was now experiencing. I strongly suspected that the problem laid in his adrenal gland, which was now secreting excess amounts of one of its hormones – probably epinephrine; and so I now had to set about proving that this was the case.

The adrenal gland sits like a cap on top of each kidney. By secreting both cortisol and epinephrine it allows us to get through stressful situations. Both hormones raise our blood pressure, and epinephrine also acts on the heart to make it work harder. These effects allow us to run away from thieves and to get through stressful events such as surgeries. For example, if a patient were to have gallbladder surgery, his or her cortisol level before the surgery might be 8 to 10. That same level measured an hour after the surgery has been performed could be as high as 35 – thereby supporting the patient in this time of stress. The amount of epinephrine secreted by the adrenal gland would also rise, in concert with the cortisol secretion.

There are a number of mechanisms by which the adrenal gland might secrete excess cortisol, thus giving rise to an increased blood pressure; however, when it comes to the release of excess epinephrine and/or norepinephrine, a tumor is most often involved; the tumor is called a pheochromocytoma, which secretes the catecholamines mentioned above.

Pheochromocytomas are rare, occurring in point-8 per 100,000 persons per year. The tumor itself is most often benign, in that it does not spread to other areas. It reeks its havoc by producing the excess hormones. Ninety percent of these tumors are located in one of the adrenal glands, but can also be located in other regions of the body – even in the bladder. Most of the time the only symptom is hypertension, since the epinephrine and norepinephrine squeeze the blood vessels throughout the body and increase the heart's contractions.

However, as the levels of these hormones rise, the patient may start to experience further symptoms, such as rising levels of hypertension, chest pain, palpitations -- because of heart irritability -- sweating, or even lightheadedness. This latter symptom develops because the high catecholamine levels in the body cause excessive fluid losses through the kidney, essentially dehydrating the victim. Some of these symptoms occur because the release of the catecholamines by the tumor may be constant but with occasional "spirts" of the hormones as well. These tumors most often do not kill patients by metastasizing but rather by accelerating the effects of hypertension, thereby producing strokes, heart attacks, and fainting spells as a result of the rapid heart rates that can occur. Fluid losses also contribute to the fainting episodes. However, the bottom line is that, if they are not diagnosed, these tumors ultimately kill people.

I strongly suspected that Eddie had a pheochromocytoma; now I had to both try to diagnose it and, additionally, control his hypertension. In order to accomplish the latter I would add a drug which would attenuate effects of the catecholamines on the blood vessels. That day I started him on Doxazosin to do just that, and ordered the appropriate hormone tests to see if I might confirm his diagnosis. I rechecked his kidney function and potassium levels, and ordered a serum catecholamine level, which would document any elevation in his levels of those hormones. Since I also had to be certain that elevated cortisol levels were not involved in his problem, I obtained a 24-hour urine specimen to assess his cortisol output.

Eddie returned for follow up in two weeks he was definitely feeling better. His home blood pressure readings were now in the normal range, and the episodes of sweating and heart palpitations were now rare. I checked his blood pressure in the office, and found it to be 122/72 – perfect.

We now turned our attention to his laboratory studies. His kidneys and potassium levels were normal, as was the 24-hour urine cortisol production. However, his level of serum catecholamines was elevated to six times the upper limit of normal. This result strongly suggested that, indeed, Eddie had a pheochromocytoma lurking somewhere in his body. I now had to find it, and then refer him to someone who could remove the tumor.

I added Metoprolol to his drug regimen in order to finish blocking all of the effects of the excess hormones, and then ordered a CT scan of his abdomen and pelvis with the addition of contrast in order to localize the tumor. My wonderfully efficient nurse was able to schedule this study for Friday – in just two days.

Eddie returned a week later to go over results. All of his symptoms had resolved, and his blood pressure readings were in the 120/68 range. This was also confirmed by my office reading as well. However, the CT scan confirmed that he indeed had a tumor. It was not in either adrenal gland, but rather was located in the nervous tissue that follows the large blood vessel (known as the aorta) that traverses the abdomen on its way to deliver blood to the legs. Lengthwise the tumor was about four inches long, with a width of about three quarters of an inch – a significant mass indeed.

So, I had found the ember which was involved Eddie's disease process. At this point the tumor must be removed in order to cure his problem. I decided to refer him to the University of Texas MD Anderson Cancer Center in Houston because its doctors have the most experience with this kind of problem. I had already initiated the necessary drug therapy which would be needed preoperatively, so that the doctors there would not have to waste time starting Eddie on those. I made the referral.

The next time I saw Eddie in my office was two weeks after the surgery had been performed. Except for some pain at the incision site (the scar was on his right flank and significantly longer than I had expected), he felt great. He was now taking only one blood pressure medicine, and his pressure readings at home were normal. All of the other symptoms were gone as well. On examination I found that his blood pressure was normal, and his wound was healing nicely. Before he left the office, I drew his serum catecholamines again, which returned a week later and were now normal.

I followed Eddie during the remainder of my time in Sweetwater, until I retired in March, 2016. Eddie had retired a few years earlier, and he and his wife now traveled quite a bit, with lots of pictures on Facebook demonstrating their happiness. Eddie's blood pressure remained well controlled, and periodic measurements of his serum catecholamine levels and CT scans continued to demonstrate the absence of tumor.

These tumors are quite rare. I found it because, in my studies over the years, I had reviewed this particular disorder many times. Sherlock always said, "If you are unaware of the existence of something then you won't know to look for it." In medicine, disorders that are rare are sometimes called "zebras." Over my forty year career in medicine, I concentrated on studying these rarer disorders so that I would be able to recognize the "zebras" lurking among the horses.

CHAPTER 4

SWEETWATER

After I left Idaho, I joined a large multispecialty group in Austin, Texas, known as the Austin Regional Clinic. Roughly about one-hundred-fifty physicians comprised this group, which was dedicated to bringing good primary care to its patients. At the time that I joined the practice there were five other I internists in the group, the rest of the physicians being mostly family practice, with three ob-gyn doctors and three general surgeons to complete the nucleus of the practice. I was assigned to work in the south clinic with another internist named Howard Marking. He was from the New York area, and had been in Austin since the beginning of the clinic, which was started by a very astute businessman named Norman Cheney – a family practice doctor who decided that, in the age of HMO's, he could start a clinic and actually make some money. And, indeed, in only about six years he had masterfully made contracts with insurance companies that had allowed him to grow the clinic to its present size. Dr. Cheney slowly thought out a problem, and then decided how he was going to solve it. I always admired him for this, and watched with amazement as he guided the group through the major changes that would occur in medicine over the coming years

I joined the clinic at a time when we, as yet, had no cell phones; being "on call" was a nightmare because we would be paged constantly by the three hospitals that we were covering. Our weekend "call" would begin Friday at six and would end Monday morning. Sleep would be an "unfamiliar friend" during those weekends. We all carried a bunch of quarters with us at all times, so that we would be able to stop at a pay phone (remember those?) and answer our pages. We would make "rounds" on our own patients that we had in the hospital as well as those of the other five internists; if anyone needed admission at any of the three hospitals that we covered, then we would do the history and physical on those patients as well. When in about 1990 I got my first cell phone, I felt like I had just fallen into "high cotton." It was a behemoth that I left plugged into the dashboard of the car at all times; but I could now get rid of all of those damned quarters.

It was the feeling of not being in control that I hated while I worked at the clinic – of being stuck in traffic when a nurse would call from one of the hospitals to tell me that a patient was going bad, and yet I would not be able to get to the hospital to assess that patient for at least another half hour or forty-five minutes. Granted, I could give the nurse some preliminary orders for the patient to be done before I arrived; but the fact that I could not physically evaluate such a patient in a matter of five to ten minutes always gave me severe anxiety.

Finally, in 1999, I decided to leave the clinic and join a group that provided "hospitalist" services to a couple of hospitals – one in South Austin and one in San Marcos, Texas – a thirty minute commute from Austin. I elected to cover the hospital in San Marcos with another internist – every other day and every other weekend "on call." When working, I stayed in the hospital, thereby being able to evaluate patients that needed admission in a timely manner as well as to manage the hospital patients without the anxiety that I had had while at the clinic. However, I discovered that, because of all of the uninsured patients that we were admitting from the ER and caring for during their hospital stay, the group was having problems collecting money -- a fact that was manifest in my paychecks. Consequently, after a few months at this job, I started looking around for another position in a small town – after all, that's really the type of practice that I enjoyed the most.

I sent my resume to a recruiting firm, which, fairly soon, came up with three possibilities: one was a teaching position at the Texas Tech Medical School in Odessa in West Texas. Now, that certainly appealed to me simply because I loved to teach. I taught at the Internal medicine residency program during my time in Austin; I was voted "Attending Physician of the Year" in 1992 by the residents in training.

Another offer was from a town in East Texas, a place where I really didn't want to live. The last was from a clinic in Sweetwater, Texas, which is a town of twelve thousand, located a forty-minute drive west from Abilene in West Texas; I decided to interview for the first and third positions.

March of 2000 found me at the medical school in Odessa. I had worn a very nice mock turtle-neck sweater, and had on good gabardine pants and a sport coat to match. Donald Lufkin, an internist, who also managed to sub-specialize in his practice to do rheumatology, was currently the head of the Internal Medicine Department; he showed me around the hospital and introduced me to all of the other members. In the ICU he presented a current case of a critically ill patient who had hip surgery and who was now in respiratory distress. I told him how I would treat the patient at this point; the main diagnostic possibilities being an acute pulmonary embolus (caused either by a blood clot or a fat embolus -- arising from the bone marrow being released into the blood at the time of surgery, or from the cement used in surgery potentially entering the bloodstream and traveling to the lungs). An acute myocardial infarction also needed to be considered. He seemed satisfied with my responses, and we finished our hospital tour.

The next morning found me hosting the "morning report" for the residents in training at the facility. In this scenario each resident who was "on call" the night before presents his or her admissions to an attending physician in order both to get a critique of the management overnight as well as to get the attending's thoughts on further care. The cases that the team presented to me were extremely complicated, with each patient having a number of disease processes complicating their management. The worst involved an alcoholic gentleman with cirrhosis, bleeding problems, fever and a change in his mental status. I carefully outlined his problems on the blackboard, and proceeded to discuss not only the ongoing disorders but also the proposed management of each. At the end of the session, all of the residents approached me and asked if I would be coming back.

Two weeks later found me interviewing in Sweetwater. Four family practice physicians established the clinic a few years before I arrived, after they had decided that a group practice would probably serve them better going forward than would the solo practices in which they had previously performed. They had added Jeremy Smola, the son of one of the family physicians, a couple of years before, and were now looking for an internist for the town. This city had a hospital district, with taxes supporting the hospital; so it would be around in the coming years.

I spent two days in Sweetwater, and liked what I saw. With two gypsum plants in town providing a lot of the employment, the economy seemed to be stable. City planners were anticipating oil and wind farm expansion in the future, which would provide more jobs. Farms and ranches spread out from the confines of the town, with cotton and cattle-ranching bringing more money into the community. I spent a number of hours talking with the members of the group, and I was impressed by how well they seemed to get along – not always the case with doctors, who sometimes have very large egos. I found the hospital to be adequate, with about thirty-five medical-surgical beds, and a five bed ICU. Radiology had CT scanning capabilities. Air ambulance transfer to larger facilities, most often to Abilene, was in place – unlike my first practice in Rupert, Idaho. I left Sweetwater on that Sunday feeling that I could easily practice here and be comfortable.

I waited for the recruiter to call me. The opportunity in Odessa intrigued me. And the fact that the Midland-Odessa area was significantly larger than Sweetwater put me off slightly, since I really wanted to be in a rural environment again. Each had its merits, only in different ways. When the recruiter called later in the week, I learned that the group in Sweetwater had made me a good offer, while Dr. Lufkin had narrowed down his choice to between me and another internist. The recruiter commented that my performance in the interview process had been superb, but that Dr. Luftkin had expressed some dismay that I had not a donned a tie for the interview.

At this point in my career I had twenty-five years of experience under my belt, and had continued to read avidly in order to keep up with changes that inevitably occur in the practice of medicine. The expertise that I had demonstrated in running the "morning report" during the interview process had certainly demonstrated that; so that the only thing that the head of the department could comment on was my lack of a tie. So I made the decision that I probably would not be a good fit at the medical school, and called the recruiter back; I would be on my way to Sweetwater in September.

It took a few months to get all my paperwork done so that the hospital could credential me. Meanwhile, my wife (I had remarried by this time) and I put the house in Austin on the market, and made a number of trips to Sweetwater in order to find a house to live in. By August everything had fallen into place. We had a contract on the house, movers had been contacted, and I had completed all of the paperwork for the hospital; we headed to Sweetwater right after Labor Day.

CHAPTER 5

NAUSEA

One of the first things that I had to do when I arrived in Sweetwater was to hire a nurse. To this end I interviewed five nurses whom the clinic thought might be appropriate. Of these, one stood out far above the rest. She was an LVN named Michelle, who had experience both in helping to run a local nursing home as well time spent working in a doctor's office. She was extremely bright, and appeared to be an assertive woman (I have always believed that the nurses who work with me should be a partner in my delivery of care to my patients – that they should be able to confront me if they thought that I was about to do something with a patient that they thought was wrong). Michelle seemed to fit that description completely, and I hired her.

Indeed, she was to prove herself to be as good as I thought she was over the next fifteen years. Her care and concern for the patients for whom we cared was genuine, and I found over the coming years that her organizational skills were absolutely amazing. We saw patients with complicated medical problems. With her help I was able to care for them efficiently and thoroughly. I could not write this book without singing Michelle's praises; upon retiring last March I found leaving her to be very bittersweet. We had helped each other to deal with a number of personal issues during our time together, and had become good friends. Of all of the office nurses that I had in my career, Michelle stands out. Many of our patients owe their lives not only to me and my expertise but also to Michelle's organizational skills in getting critical lab work or radiologic procedures done in a timely manner so that I might treat them properly. I could not have asked for a better partner during my years in Sweetwater.

As the local internist one of the things that I did for the other physicians in the community was to consult on their complicated cases about which they had questions in diagnosis or management. In rural medicine, cooperation among doctors makes possible a level of care for patients unavailable without the insight of several physicians. This service might involve seeing their patient when he or she was in the hospital or scheduling office consultation time so that I might evaluate them there.

One of the most interesting patients referred to me during my time in Sweetwater was a man of seventy-four who had presented to his family physician with a complaint of intermittent nausea. The nausea had caused his primary MD to hospitalize him for further management. After much testing, his doctor and the surgical consultant thought that his gallbladder may be the culprit; so the patient underwent a cholecystectomy. However, now three days post-op, the patient was still having symptoms. It was at this point that his primary physician asked me to see him in consultation. I had my first visit with Mr. Lawrence Wells later that same evening in his hospital room. However, before I discuss Mr. Well's problem further, I would like to digress for a while to explain what is involved in performing a consultation such as that which I was about to do on this patient.

The first thing that I do as I begin the consultative process is to review the patient's chart so that I AM familiar with everything that has gone on up to this point in time. This review includes going over all of the laboratory results and radiologic results that have been ordered by his previous treating physicians. This review most often involves a perusal of all of the patient's charts from his or her prior admissions to the hospital as well, as I look for clues in the previously dictated histories, examinations, and lab and x-ray data. After I accomplish this task, I then must sit down with the patient and his family and take from them a very detailed history of the present problem – starting from the very beginning of any symptoms. Aside from the review of the chart noted above, this part of the consultation (or any patient encounter, for that matter) is THE most important part of the process. It is in the history of the present illness that the patient and/or family members give me extremely important clues concerning the progression of the disease process, thus alerting me to the presence of "embers" in that progression. Obviously, in order to make sense out of the many symptoms that might be presented to me during this part of the evaluation, I needed to have a very good working knowledge of how both common and uncommon diseases might affect a patient, which allows me to narrow down the number of potential diagnoses. As we progress through the history I AM mentally checking off which disorders do and don't fit as a possibility. The process continues as I review every system in the body with the patient; so that, before I ever lay a hand on this person to examine him, I will have narrowed the possible disorders potentially present to just three or four – always reminding myself that this human being may have both "ticks and fleas" -- meaning that there may be more than one disease process occurring in this person.

I next do a physical examination on the patient, looking for any evidence supporting my tentative diagnoses as well as further evidence to rule out other possibilities. If that person has a known chronic disease such as diabetes, I will also be looking in my exam for evidence of complications of that disease, such as signs of heart disease or a problem with their circulation. Problems with the person's nervous system would dictate that I do a complete neurologic exam on that patient as well. Thus, after obtaining the history, I might take anywhere from twenty minutes to forty-five minutes to do an adequate exam.

These steps concluded, I then sit down with the patient and family members to discuss my findings, probable diagnoses, and tests that I might need in order to confirm my thought processes. I explain to them very carefully how I arrived at my conclusions, and answer any questions that anyone has. Finally, after dictating my consultation note (which might take another twenty minutes), I call the referring doctor to let him know what I AM thinking and what tests I AM ordering to further solidify my diagnoses. Ah, but now I return to Mr. Wells and his problem.

Mr. Wells was a seventy-four year old man who had been perfectly healthy until about five months previous to my examination, when he developed episodes of nausea. The attacks would occur from six to fifteen times a day, and would last anywhere from ten to twenty seconds. What was a bit unusual about his symptoms was that he lacked any associated symptoms of abdominal pain, fever, chills, actual vomiting, or any problems with gastrointestinal bleeding. He had lost about fifteen pounds over the last five months because of his symptoms. However, what also concerned the family was the patient's significant loss of memory over the period of his illness. In fact, this was such a problem that Mr. Wells could not provide me with all of the details of his illness over the last months, and I had to query the family members about those.

After forty-five minutes spent in history-taking, I was now ready to examine Mr. Wells. I finally asked the most critical question of all: "Can you communicate with the patient during his episodes?" The answer "No," provided me with THE most informative clue about his disorder – namely that Mr. Wells was briefly disengaged from his environment during his "spells." I now certainly had at least part of the diagnosis. And so I began his examination …

On general examination, Mr. Wells appeared to be very healthy. He was tall, about six feet, with a full crop of grey hair. He spoke normally and moved around the exam room without any difficulty. His vital signs were normal. My examination of his cardiovascular system revealed no problems, and his abdomen was without tenderness to my palpation except at his recent incision. Prior rectal exams had shown no masses or evidence of GI bleeding, so I did not now repeat that. My examination of his testicles revealed no masses. I found no evidence of enlarged lymph glands which might suggest a malignancy. I now focused on his neurological exam.

Other than the fact that he felt nauseated at times, Mr. Wells could not tell me much else about his trouble, yet he knew the date, time, location, and could understand me and follow commands easily. His reading ability was not impaired, nor did he demonstrate any focal weakness of arm or leg that might suggest a prior stroke. I found his coordination to be normal. However, he was not able to recall three numbers that I had given him five minutes ago. I did a careful examination of all of his senses – they were also normal. I had just completed my examination and was washing my hands, when his wife said "Look. He is having another episode."

Indeed, the patient was now changed from just a few seconds ago. His head was turned slightly to the right and he stared blankly at the wall. He did not respond to me when I called his name; nothing else was different. It was all over in about fifteen seconds, after which Mr. Wells regained his normality over the next three to four minutes. I now was certain of at least one of my diagnoses – Mr. Wells was having partial seizures.

We are all familiar with what is known as a "grand mal" seizure, in which the patient falls to the ground, thrashing around and foaming at the mouth – all of which might last from thirty seconds up to a couple of minutes. This phenomenon is truly quite scary, and represents an "electrical storm" that is occurring in that person's brain. During a seizure like this, the patient can't breathe; so that, if the seizure doesn't stop, the brain suffers irreversible damage as it continues the "storm" without an adequate oxygen supply. The electrical discharges usually begin on one side of the brain and then spread to involve the entire brain neuronal tissue; so that the patient loses consciousness during the episode. There are multiple causes of seizures, among which are prior head injury, infection, stroke, or brain hemorrhage. Other causes include autoimmune diseases, in which the body attacks its own tissues in different areas – the brain included. In a significant number of patients we find NO structural lesion in the brain that might initiate the onset of seizure activity. These persons have "primary epilepsy."

In some cases, however, the "storm" remains localized to just one part of the brain, thus giving rise to "focal seizures." These often last only a few seconds, during which time the person is still disconnected mentally from his environment and is unable to communicate with anyone – just like the patient with a "grand mal" episode. One can see then that, if these episodes occur often enough during the day, the overall electrical functioning of the subject's brain might be disturbed, thereby producing learning disabilities or memory problems.

The type of seizure of which I speak often is localized to the "temporal lobe" of the brain – a region in which memories are stored and retrieved. Patients who have these partial seizure episodes will suffer brief periods of seizure activity localized to that area; if multiple episodes happen during a twenty-four hour period, the disturbances in the temporal lobe will impair memory formation and recall. I was convinced now that Mr. Wells was having enough focal seizure activity during the day that the frequency of this activity foiled his brain's ability to process memories. (He could not communicate to me any memories about the last five months.) As some people experience different odors during this type of epilepsy, this patient was experiencing nausea. Nausea arising from the stomach, intestine or gallbladder disease does not stop in just a few seconds; that type of nausea may go on for hours. I was now certain that the brief episodes of nausea that Mr. Wells was experiencing were surely arising from abnormal brain discharges.

I had reviewed all of his charts with their accumulated data before I entered the patient's room. Yes, he had a few small gallstones found on ultrasound examination; however, after obtaining his history, I was convinced that these were merely "hanging out" and were causing Mr. Wells no problem. A CT scan of his abdomen and pelvis had also been normal pre-operatively. His routine blood tests were absolutely normal.

So now I had a working diagnosis: temporal lobe epilepsy, which would explain his symptom complex. I now had to document his disorder with an EEG (a brain-wave test) and search for a possible cause of the problem. An EEG done the following day did, indeed, show abnormal electrical firing located in the left temporal lobe. I started the patient on Tegretol and Lamictal – antiepileptic medications which are excellent for controlling discharges in that region of the brain. The following Thursday Mr. Wells underwent brain imaging with an MRI, with intravenous contrast given in order to visualize the different parts of his brain more completely. Additionally, I ordered ultrasound imaging of his carotid arteries to check on the blood supply to his brain and drew multiple blood samples in order to help sort through the various potential causes for his problem. He and his wife were to return for follow up on the next Tuesday. Pending the blood test results, I started him on Thiamine – a vitamin vitally necessary for the functioning of the brain, especially that part involved in memory.

The brain is truly a miraculous organ. Billions of neuron cells are organized into many different functional regions, an organization which allows us to deal with our different environments. Our brains allow us to have a concept of "self." Although the neuronal cells "fire" electrically, communication between each cell is accomplished via the release of chemical neurotransmitters from the ends of the axon of the cell. These chemicals then traverse a minute space and enter the axon or axons of neighboring cells – thereby allowing us to analyze situations, learn new things, and carry out complex physical activities.

Imagine for a minute a pole-vaulter standing at the end of the runway, about to begin his vault at a height of fifteen feet. He stands silently for a few minutes while, with the frontal lobes of his brain, he analyzes the wind speed, the speed of his run up that he feels he needs in order to clear the bar, and goes over in his mind all of the different movements needed in order to succeed. Finally, he begins his run, carrying a heavy pole which he needs to plant at precisely the right time so that he can leave the ground and ascend skyward. Now the motor part of his brain along with the cerebellum (the coordination center) has taken over. We watch our vaulter as he gains speed, all the while gradually lowering the pole until he ultimately plants the far end of the device into the box and thus begins his ascent toward the bar. The motor strip and the cerebellum continue to "fire," allowing him to execute all of the maneuvers that he has practiced so often – the motor patterns that his brain has, hopefully, integrated successfully. Quite a feat – all accomplished because of the brain's electrical and chemical communication ability.

Our brain functioning allows us to develop language skills, to learn about our universe, to protect ourselves from threats, to hold treasured memories within our temporal lobe, and, thanks to the functioning of the amygdala located near the temporal lobe, to have loving relationships with one another. The brain is the organ of our "being," our "selfness." When the thinking part of the brain finally dies, so do we – even though some of our other organs may continue to function for a while because of the automaticity of the heart and other organs.

Our brains may sustain injuries in many different ways. As we all know from reading the news and watching TV, blunt force trauma to the skull may damage the underlying brain tissue to the point where it is no longer viable. In this instance the brain is not only directly damaged, but the swelling produced by the local damage ultimately raises pressure inside of the skull to the point where the remainder of the brain loses its blood supply and therefore dies. Infections such as West Nile Virus along with other viruses can produce enough inflammation in the brain neurons that they can no longer function. A stroke, caused either by a brain bleed or the occlusion of blood vessels supplying a part of the brain will produce a devastating loss of brain cells, with subsequent severe physical impairment or even death. Many are familiar with someone who has had a brain tumor, which often does not respond well to treatments. Such a mass encroaches on the rest of the brain cells and raises the pressure inside of the skull until the patient finally succumbs to its effects. Infections such as syphilis or tuberculosis will, ultimately, infect the brain if left untreated. Lastly, autoimmune diseases, disorders in which the body attacks its own tissues, also cause dysfunction of nervous tissue. Systemic lupus is the prototype of this form of illness; in the brain it can cause strokes, seizures, psychotic episodes, anxiety and depression. However, lupus also tends to attack other organ systems at the same time that it affects the brain – thereby signaling its presence to clinicians.

Mr. Wells and his family returned to see me in the office on the Tuesday following his MRI scan. Both he and his family were ecstatic because he had had no further "spells." His wife told me that Mr. Wells was now able to carry on conversations much better, and that his memory had improved – although he still could not remember any details of the last five months.

I now discussed the laboratory and MRI findings with them. The testing for viruses, syphilis, and lupus were all negative for any activity, and his thiamine and B12 levels were normal. The carotid study revealed that he had excellent circulation to his brain. However, I now revealed to them that the MRI was abnormal in that the left hippocampus (a region next to the left temporal lobe) had shown intense activity after the contrast had been injected into his body; the remainder of his brain appeared normal.

There are a couple of diseases that will "light up" the hippocampus on the MRI scan, as was seen on Mr. Wells' study: "Herpes encephalitis" is an acute viral infection of the brain, which rapidly renders its victim both febrile and comatose. It has a predilection for the temporal lobes, so that they may intensely take up the intravenous contrast used for MRI studies. Certainly this was not the course exhibited by Mr. Wells because his disease slowly progressed.

However, the other disorder fit both the MRI findings as well as Mr. Wells' disease progression to a "T." I speak of a rare autoimmune disease of the brain known as "limbic encephalitis." (The limbic system of the brain refers to the temporal lobe, the hippocampus, and the amygdala, the areas of our brain that are involved with memories and emotions.) The bodies of patients who develop limbic encephalitis manufacture antibodies which then attack the neurons of the brain, causing them to malfunction. These antibodies have a predilection for the neurons located within the limbic system of the brain – thus the patient's gradual presentation with memory difficulties, focal seizures, confusion or a combination of those symptoms. Such patients may be misdiagnosed as having dementia because of their inability both to form new memories and to retrieve old ones. However, unlike dementia patients, who worsen over a period of years, the progression of "limbic encephalitis" occurs over a matter of months.

Like epilepsy, limbic encephalitis may be primary or secondary to something like a brain tumor. In the first case the patient's body manufactures antibodies to different parts of the neurons for no particular reason. In secondary limbic encephalitis patients harbors a tumor somewhere in their bodies. When their bodies make antibodies against the underlying tumor, those antibodies cross react with parts of the patient's brain neurons, causing them to malfunction. To complicate matters, the underlying tumor may be undiscoverable at the time that the brain phenomenon is going on. The neurons primarily involved are located in the temporal lobe area; however, the antibodies can attack other parts of the brain as well. So far, the "paraneoplastic" blood panel that I drew from Mr. Wells at the time of his MRI had shown no obvious antibodies in the serum; however, his spinal fluid would also have to be tested for these as well.

In Mr. Wells' case, there was no evidence that he had a tumor at the time of this investigation. I found that he had had a normal chest x-ray before his operation, and his pre-operative CT scan of his abdomen and pelvis revealed no tumor in his pancreas, liver, or kidneys. He had had a normal colonoscopy just eight months before I saw him. A normal urinalysis suggested that his bladder was normal, and a PSA was in the normal range. His testicular exam had been normal.

I now explained to Mr. Wells and his family that I was certain that he had limbic encephalitis," even though the disorder is rare. I explained that, even though I had his seizures under good control, he needed to see a neurologist – both so that the specialist could confirm my diagnosis and so that he might do a spinal tap to test the spinal fluid for evidence of brain inflammation, viral infection, and for the different antibodies that could be involved in his disease. I referred Mr. Wells to Dr. Chris Vanderbilt, my favorite neurologist at Shannon Clinic in San Angelo, Texas, who saw him the following day.

Dr. Vanderbilt accomplished the spinal tap and sent the fluid for all of the necessary studies. He also repeated the MRI, just to confirm my findings. In the end, he agreed with my diagnosis, continued the antiepileptic drugs that I had started, and began Mr. Wells on a course of high-dose steroids intravenously to cut down on the antibody production by Mr. Wells' body. The spinal fluid studies showed evidence for mild inflammation, with an elevated protein count, but was negative for all viruses as well as for antibodies that are commonly involved in this particular disorder. Lastly, the pathologist found no tumor cells in the spinal fluid.

About this time family members in Dallas called San Angelo to demand that Mr. Wells be transferred to a neurologist of their choice in the Dallas area; obviously they could not believe that physicians in smaller communities might even remotely arrive at the correct diagnosis and treatment for their father.

And so Mr. Wells was transferred to the neurologist in Dallas, who reviewed all of the studies that we had performed, examined the patient, and confirmed our diagnosis. Following his four high-dose steroid injections there, Mr. Wells was returned to Sweetwater on the same antiepileptic drugs on which I had placed him.

I saw him back in the office for follow up two weeks later, at which time he was feeling great. His nausea was gone, and he had gained back five pounds in weight. His wife had noticed no "spells;" he had even headed back to the golf course.

I followed Mr. Wells until I retired in March, 2015. During that follow up period, he had one flair-up of his disease activity, which the neurologist treated with another burst of intravenous steroids. Repeat exams, lab work, and x-rays have thus far revealed no evidence for an underlying tumor.

Such cases as Mr. Wells are indeed rare. As his history indicated, the disease that afflicted him smoldered for a while before it began to present other clues. In a town the size of Sweetwater I was able to make the diagnosis because I had read case reports of it in the *New England Journal of Medicine*, a journal that I perused every weekend. I didn't have to wear a suit and tie and live in a metropolitan area in order to read that publication. With the help of that journal, and by following the axiom "If you listen to the patient long enough they will tell you what is wrong with them," I was able to follow the embers in this case as they began to spread, and, by so doing, make a diagnosis. In Sweetwater, I was to see patients who had other rare diseases, some of which had smoldered for a number of years before I ultimately saw the patient and made a diagnosis.

CHAPTER 6

A YOUNG WOMAN WITH
ABDOMINAL PAIN

W hen I was a medical student at Loyola-Stritch Medical School in Chicago I had a couple of jobs. In my third year I was lucky enough to be chosen to work in the medical library at the VA hospital located at Hines, Illinois, which was located about the length of a football field from the medical school. Working there provided me with room and board in the VA campus housing --a gift that I found to be very helpful, given my limited resources. In the library I checked out medical books to the medical students and residents, and then filed them back on the shelves when they returned the books.

Often business was slow in the library, and I was able to study as I waited for people to arrive; and, during these slow times, I was able to peruse many of the textbooks that I found there. It was during one of these times that I stumbled upon a book which shaped my approach to the practice of medicine for the rest of my career. This gem was *Hamilton Bailey's Demonstration of Physical Signs in Clinical Surgery*, a book about physical diagnosis written by a renowned English surgeon. He was born in the early 1900's, and died about 1949. He wrote this book at a time when CT and MRI scanners did not exist, so that the taking of an accurate history along with expertise in the physical examination of the patient by the attending physician were absolutely necessary if that physician were to arrive at a correct diagnosis. In reading this book I found innumerable "pearls" about the physical examination of the patient – information that I immediately began to apply in the examination of patients that I encountered. Indeed, this book influenced my practice of medicine for the next forty years. I re-read it many times over that period, and even dictated many of the chapters on tape so that I could listen to them while I drove, thus refreshing my memory about certain physical findings in patients. I have read many other books about physical examination over my career; however, Hamilton Bailey's book on the subject has, in my mind, remained the "gold standard" of this genre. In my career in medicine I have always taught either medical students or residents; my mantra to them has always been, "When all else fails, take a history and examine the patient." Even though the government would like to take away our ability to document an accurate history and exam by its "click the box" approach to these aspects of medicine while, at the same time, it takes away our valuable time with each patient by forcing us to use these electronic record systems, an accurate history from and physical examination of the patient remain today, as in Hamilton Bailey's time, the cornerstones for the practice of good medicine. And so, as I begin this chapter, I offer a quotation from Dr. Bailey concerning the examination of a patient with acute abdominal pain: "Physical signs and their interpretation reach a high pinnacle of importance in the diagnosis of acute abdominal disease. Frequently and urgent an all-important decision has to be reached by their aid alone. It is for this reason that no section of this book rivals this in responsibility." I now come to the next case.

Erica Gerhard was a woman in her late twenties when I was asked by her attending physician to consult on her in the hospital. She had been admitted with abdominal pain, and had undergone an esophagogastroenteroscopy a colonoscopy, and even an abdominal exploratory surgery with removal of her gallbladder. Now, six days postoperatively, she was still having the same pain that had brought her into the hospital; I was asked to see her. By collecting her detailed history, I soon became aware that her disease had been smoldering for many years. Periodically it would erupt into an acute episode – episodes that were often triggered by attempts to medicate her; the disorder had not only affected her abdomen over those years, but her nervous system as well. It seemed to be a systemic problem.

Erica is about five-feet four inches tall, one hundred and fifty pounds, with brown hair and eyes. It was obvious to me that she was still in pain. As she now sat on the edge of her bed, she narrated her history to me: Erica had become depressed about age twelve. Her doctors had prescribed many different antidepressant medications over the next few years; however, at age sixteen she was hospitalized in a psychiatric unit because of suicidal thoughts. New medications were prescribed, and she improved enough that, by age eighteen, she was able to go to Norway for a while. While she was there, she felt much better, and stopped all of her medications; even after doing so, Erica continued to do well. She told me that, while in Norway, she had been on a high-carbohydrate diet, and had gained a little weight; and, mentally and physically she felt good.

Erica returned to the states and started college. However, within a short time her severe depressive symptoms returned. Hospitalized at a psychiatric unit again, multiple antidepressants were again started by her physicians; they even started her on antipsychotic medication as well – diagnosing her as having depression with psychotic tendencies.

This sort of "psychiatric cycle" continued, and Erica ultimately spent a month at Big Spring State Hospital at age twenty one, diagnosed as "bipolar" and "borderline personality disorder." She told me that during her time at the State Hospital the physicians changed her medications almost weekly. However, after her discharge from that facility, she went back to college and finally finished her degree – in spite of being on many different medications for her psychiatric problems during that time. On one occasion during these times, she was hospitalized with acute urinary retention and abdominal pain, which resolved after her physicians withheld her medications.

After graduating, Erica found that she could not seem to hold a job for longer than about three months at a time because, as she would tell me, "I would mentally lose it." In 2005, her clinician changed her medication "cocktail" to the combination of Abilify (a new antipsychotic drug), Topamax (an antiepileptic medication), and Wellbutrin (an antidepressant).

Shortly after this last medication change Erica developed serious problems; she developed severe right upper quadrant abdominal pain, severe constipation, and difficulty urinating. Although she was living in San Angelo at the time, she decided to see a physician in Sweetwater because her mother was a nurse working at Rolling Plains Memorial Hospital in our town. She had been admitted, and underwent the procedures that I have noted. Her consulting surgeon was even talking with her about performing a total colectomy surgery on her because of her inability to have a bowel movement.

As I listened to her history, I felt that this poor woman's disease had been smoldering for years, manifesting itself in her psychiatric symptoms. However, those embers had now spread to the point where the disorder was demonstrating its other symptoms in this patient, leading to both the former hospitalization and to this one.

Although she had severe right upper quadrant pain, this pain was not associated with fever, chills, chest pain, cough, or radiation to her back or shoulder. Although she experienced nausea, she had not been vomiting. She did not drink alcohol, nor did she use any "street drugs." She suffered from occasional headaches, but had never had any seizures or any focal weakness of her arms or legs. She had never had any problems with her skin. My review of her chart and x-rays prior to visiting with her had shown that she had only a slight elevation of her white blood cell count, normal liver and kidney function tests, and a normal urinalysis; the CT scan of her abdomen revealed only constipation. Her pancreas enzymes in the blood were in the normal range, and the pancreas appeared normal on the CT. Her gallbladder sonogram showed only a little "sludge," but no stones or thickening of the gallbladder wall; the latter would indicate inflammation of that organ. The blood sedimentation rate (a measure of inflammation) was also in the normal range.

As I listened to Erica tell me about her illness, my heart began to beat a little more quickly, and I became agitated with excitement. The hair on the back of my neck stood up and my eyes widened as I listened to every twist and turn of this poor woman's disease process. Indeed, I had read this story many times in the journals and textbooks that I had studied over the years, and had looked for this illness in many, many patients presenting to me over the years with symptoms of abdominal pain. Even so, I had never diagnosed this disease previously in my career. I was now about to do so; by the time that I had taken her complete history, I knew her diagnosis. I proceeded with my examination.

At the time of my examination, Erica's vital signs were normal. Examination of her head, neck, heart, and lungs was normal. However, my examination of her abdomen revealed that she still had marked tenderness to even gentle palpation of the right side of her abdomen, while the left side was really not tender at all. A manual pelvic and rectal exam showed only some stool in the rectum; the uterus was not tender when I moved it. I found no skin lesions on her body, and her joints were not tender as I palpated them. I now turned my attention to the neurologic examination.

Erica certainly seemed depressed; other than that, the examination of her mental status was normal. I examined her cranial nerves, her muscle strength in the arms and legs, and I discovered normal findings. However, I found absolutely no tendon reflexes at her Achilles tendons, and her ability to discern a pinprick on the skin of both feet was markedly diminished – both findings indicating a problem with her peripheral nerves, and findings that are definitely abnormal in a woman of her age.

In most of us who develop severe abdominal pain our first thought becomes "AM I going to need surgery for this?" Indeed, when I as a physician examine a patient with acute, severe abdominal pain, I have to ask the same question: "Does this particular patient need an operation?" Certainly, there are disorders that can only be solved by surgery, such as acute appendicitis, acute cholecystitis, and perforation of the stomach or intestine. However, the list of disorders that can cause a patient to have severe abdominal pain is exceedingly long; so that a physician must take a very detailed history from the patient in order that he or she might recognize a "disease pattern" in that history that suggests a clue to the correct diagnosis. In Erica's case the clues concerning her real diagnosis were revealed in the history of her psychiatric symptoms together with the emergence of her abdominal symptoms on two occasions, the last episode beginning with her recent changes in her psychiatric medications. My neurologic exam also suggested another clue, with her absent reflexes at the ankles and her difficulty with sensation in her feet.

In Erica's case there exists a deficiency of an enzyme that is involved in her cells that make hemoglobin – the molecule that is located in our red blood cells to which oxygen binds, and which is thereby delivered to all of our tissues. This enzyme (porphobilinogen deaminase) is located in the middle of the molecular cascade involved in the production of heme, the molecule to which iron is attached in order to form hemoglobin. The hemoglobin is then inserted into our red blood cells so that they might carry oxygen to our tissues. Most patients with this disorder have only about fifty percent activity of this enzyme.

At the beginning of the cascade resides the enzyme ALA synthase, an enzyme that facilitates the union of glycine and succinyl-coenzyme A to form delta 5 aminolevulinic acid (ALA) -- the first molecule in the Heme - formation sequence. If the activity of this first enzyme is increased (which can occur with many different medications, with fasting, or with many different kinds of stress) then ALA levels increase because of the enzyme deficiency that is present further downstream.

ALA happens to be structurally very similar to gamma-aminobutyric acid (GABA), which is THE major inhibitory neurotransmitter throughout our nervous system – including both the brain and the peripheral nervous system. Therefore, when ALA accumulates in excess amounts, as it does in Erica's disease, it occupies the GABA receptors on nervous tissue and inhibits functioning of the brain and of the peripheral nerves. In the brain this inhibition produces all kinds of psychiatric symptoms, and even effects changes that can be visualized on MRI scanning – which was demonstrated in the patient afflicted with this disorder discussed in Case 20-2008 in the *New England Journal of Medicine*. When imaged by MRI, the brain of that patient showed hyper-intensity in many of its areas when contrast was administered. The radiologists interpreted this and other findings on the MRI as representing a reversible abnormality of the brain.

The inhibition of peripheral nerve activity by the excess ALA accumulation affects both our autonomic nervous system as well as peripheral nerves that go to our extremities, which allow both motion and sensation in those extremities. Inhibition of activity in the autonomic nervous system produces neurogenic abdominal pain, constipation, inhibition of urination, and can also effect changes in our pulse and blood pressure. Inhibition of the other peripheral nerves can produce muscular paralysis in a patient – even to the point of paralysis of respiratory muscles, so that the patient has to be intubated and placed on a respirator. More commonly, however, the inhibition of these nerves will affect the patient's sensory abilities; the loss of Erica's reflex at her ankle, along with the sensory deficit that I had found in her feet certainly confirmed that she had involvement of her peripheral nerves. Her retention of urine and constipation indicated that her autonomic nervous system was also compromised by this disease process.

So what is this disease that had been complicating Erica's life ever since she was a teenager? The embers were present even back then, and continued to smolder within her until this final change in her medications had dramatically Induced increased activity of the ALA synthase, and thus the levels of ALA. The disorder is called Acute Intermittent Porphyria, and is caused by a mutation in a gene, which lowers the levels of the enzyme porphobilinogen deaminase – that enzyme located in the middle of the heme production cascade. With a decrease in heme production, there is an even further increase in ALA, since the end product heme is now too low to effect suppression of that initiating enzyme.   And so, once there is stimulation of ALA synthase, a vicious cycle begins, which will continue until enough heme is given to the patient to "turn off" that particular enzyme.

So, from Erica's history I was fairly confident that she had Acute Intermittent Porphyria. I had to consider other problems, such as adrenal insufficiency, heavy metal poisoning, and Hereditary Angioedema – all of which can cause severe abdominal pain. I therefore tested her morning cortisol level, which returned at 18 micrograms/deciliter – a normal value consistent with her level of stress. The other tests also returned in the normal range. I measured the level of ALA and porphobilinogen in her body, and collected a twenty-four hour urine, again looking for an excess level; but now I also had to treat her.

As I mentioned above, heme, when made in normal amounts, feeds back on the enzyme ALA synthase, so that the levels of ALA do not rise above normal levels. So the treatment for Erica at this time was straightforward: I have to give her the heme that her body was lacking in order to turn off the enzyme.

Since this disease is rare, most hospitals (including our small one) don't generally stock Panhematin (the trade name for the heme drug) in their pharmacies. It took two days for us to finally get the medication; I then started Erica on the treatment regimen – one vial of Panhematin intravenously daily until symptoms resolve. A typical treatment course is from four to fourteen days.

After the second dose of the drug Erica began to feel better. Her abdominal pain and nausea began to improve, and she was able to start oral intake. By day five of her treatment with Panhematin, she was now pain free. She tolerated a regular diet; and, after I had her bladder catheter removed, she was able to urinate on her own. She had received a total of four doses of the drug, and was now symptom-free as regards her abdominal pain, constipation, and inability to urinate. I had withheld all of her psychiatric drugs; but even her depression improved as we administered the Panhematin.

It would be a while yet before all the lab tests would return in order to solidify the diagnosis; however, Erica had responded dramatically to treatment with Panhematin – a medication that treats no disease other than Porphyria. I was now even more certain about her diagnosis than I had been before the treatment. But I now had to map out a plan that would hopefully keep her disease under control and diminish the number of exacerbations that she might experience.

I had the dietician instruct her about a high carbohydrate diet; the dietician stressed the fact that Erica had to eat regularly, since fasting ends up stimulating the activity of the enzyme that begins the acute attacks. I had the surgeon place an IV port under her skin, and arranged with the local pharmacist to provide Erica with a supply of dextrose solution, which she would administer as soon as she felt any abdominal pain, since the extra carbohydrate in the fluid will often abort an attack. With all of this now accomplished, I finally discharged Erica, with instructions to see me in two weeks. I did not send her home with any psychiatric drugs.

When I saw Erica back in the office at her two-week visit, she told me that she was feeling great. She indicated that she was not feeling depressed, and that she had had no further abdominal pain or nausea. She had not had to administer any of the IV dextrose so far.

I reviewed her final laboratory reports with her. Two of them were equivocal, but one certainly suggested that she indeed had Porphyria. I questioned her further about her family history: neither of her parents had had any of the symptoms that she had demonstrated; however, she seemed to recall that a great grandmother had suffered recurrent episodes of abdominal pain. I decided to continue the current management, and thereafter followed her at regular three-month intervals.

Over the next ten years, Erica had intermittent attacks of her symptoms. Some of these she was able to abort with the IV dextrose and pain medication; while, at other times, I had to admit her and treat her with the IV Panhematin. On each of those admissions her symptoms were always the same: abdominal pain, nausea, acute urinary retention, and constipation –all of which would resolve after the fourth dose of the drug. Many of these exacerbations were precipitated by the hormonal changes that would occur near the onset of her menses; so I had an OB-Gyn specialist consult with her. Finally, because of the fairly frequent peri-menstrual attacks, Erica elected to have a complete hysterectomy. That made a great difference. After that procedure I rarely had to hospitalize her for the acute episodes. Erica's sensory neuropathy symptoms worsened a bit over the years. A neurology consultant evaluated her and ruled out other causes for her peripheral nerve symptoms, agreeing that it was due to the Porphyria.

After her hysterectomy, her acute episodes diminished significantly. She and her family moved to Lubbock, Texas, which is about a two-hour drive from Sweetwater. However, she had great difficulty finding a physician there who was familiar with the disease, and who could manage her. Therefore she continued seeing me until I retired in March, 2015. She has held a steady job as a nurse in Lubbock, and has been going to school to further her education so that she can work as a psychiatric nurse. I spoke with her just before I began to write this chapter: she has found an internist in Lubbock who has another patient with Porphyria, and so is familiar with the disease and its manifestations. Erica continues on the treatment that I initially outlined for her; and, with confidence now in her new physician, I believe that she will do well. She remains off any major psychiatric drugs.

And so, once again, we have seen the embers of a disease process smolder over a very prolonged period of time before they enlarge to the point where the flames become more visible to the clinician. We will observe this phenomenon again in further cases.

CHAPTER 7

AN INTERESTING FACE

I remember that it was on a Thursday afternoon when I first saw Richard. I had already seen a couple of my patients who were scheduled for the afternoon, and I had left one of their charts on my office desk. I was heading up the hallway to consult with my next patient when I passed him going in the opposite direction. I estimated that this man was probably in his mid-sixties, around five feet seven inches tall, and weighed, probably, about one hundred eighty pounds. He wore jeans and an olive-colored shirt. He had a full head of hair, but that was not the most remarkable thing about this man's appearance.

I had taken about three steps beyond him on the way to my next exam room, when I suddenly stopped in my tracks: "That face," I said to myself, "I have seen that face before." Because I still had five patients to see that afternoon, I couldn't spend any more time wondering about the mystery at that time. However, in those few seconds that patient's face entered my temporal lobe, and the latter began its search for a match. Two or three more steps brought me to the examination room; I knocked, and then entered to begin my session with Mrs. Wayne.

It was five forty-five when I finally finished seeing my last patient for the day, and began dictating my patient notes for the day. After that, I began answering questions that had been forwarded to my computer, finally finishing up around eight PM. I then headed over to the ICU to make evening rounds on the two patients that I was managing there: One was a sixty-four-year-old woman with an exacerbation of her emphysema (but would she quit smoking – no.);

the second was a fifty-year-old gentleman who had developed inflammation of his pancreas (pancreatitis), which was caused by one of his diabetic medications. The inflammation in the pancreas basically produces a second degree burn of the tissues of the pancreas and the surrounding areas so that fluid weeps from those inflamed sites. The patient develops a rapid heart rate, a drop in blood pressure (sometimes even down to shock levels of 80/40), a reduced urine output because of the low blood pressure, and an alteration in his ability to think properly because of the low blood flow to the brain (findings very similar to those described previously in my discussion of anaphylaxis, except that they developed via a different mechanism). Therefore, the physician must be meticulous in his or her management of the patient's abdominal pain, the assessment of fluid balances, the evaluation of the patient's lungs and mental state, and the interpretations of all of the laboratory values -- all of which are needed in order to try to stabilize such a patient. If these parameters are not attended to properly (especially the fluid management), the patient's shock state may lead to the failure of the vital organs, and ultimately to his or her death. Thus, I spent another forty-five minutes just dealing with this last patient before finally saying, "Goodnight" to the ICU nurses and headed for home. I was in my car and driving the short distance to my home, when I was staring at "the face" once again. "My God!" I said to myself as I turned onto Grand Avenue; I have seen that face many times –"but where? "

I noticed that this gentleman appeared to be normal as far as his overall build was concerned. He still had a head of full grey hair, which, although it covered his pate adequately, appeared to me to be very fine. It covered his forehead almost to his eyes. He had blue eyes; however, instead of the usual type of laugh lines at the corners of each eye – lines which are normally somewhat deepened because of age and sun exposure – this man had very superficial lines that were very fine. In fact, his laugh lines were almost imperceptible. The skin over the remainder of his face was similarly thin and slightly tanned, a fact which made him look much younger than his probable age. I noticed no scars, loss of pigment in the skin, or any areas of excess pigment formation. He had no enlargement of his cheeks, which would suggest the presence of excess Cortisol secretion by his adrenal gland.

I had never seen this man in the clinic before; however, he obviously was a patient of one of my colleagues practicing there. As I pondered the appearance of this man's facial features, racking my brain for any association, the light in my brain's temporal lobe (which forms part of our memory center) finally turned on. I had, in fact, seen this face in many textbooks and medical articles on numerous occasions over the years – starting when I was a third-year medical student, perusing *Hamilton Bailey's Demonstration of Physical Signs in Clinical Surgery* in the library at the VA hospital. The face that this person in the book presented to the world demonstrated features that are classically seen in a patient who has hypopituitarism – a medical condition in which the pituitary gland is not producing some or all of the hormones that it is supposed to manufacture and secrete in order to govern all of the other glands under its control. Since that third year in medical school, I had seen almost the exact same face in many textbooks and medical journal articles in which authors were discussing hypopituitarism – its diagnosis and management. However, I had never observed a person with that face walking by me in the hallway of my clinic.

So now I had to wonder which doctor was caring for this man, and whether any tests had been run to diagnose his problem; for I was absolutely certain that this individual definitely had hypopituitarism. The next morning I questioned my nurse Michelle (a woman who knows almost everyone in Sweetwater as well as everything that goes on in our small town – and especially everything that happens in our clinic). Later in the afternoon, she was able to tell me that the patient's name was Richard Snellen, who had been seeing Dr. Luther Martin, a good family physician, complaining of various complaints for the last six months. These complaints indicated that he was predominantly feeling fatigued and had shortness of breath.

Friday was Dr. Martin's day off; so it would be Monday before I could discuss Mr. Snellen with him. I was on call over this upcoming weekend, and was busy enough that I had no time to again mull over Mr. Snellen and his potential problems.

I arrived at the clinic Monday at 10 AM after making my rounds at the hospital. Michelle called me over to the computer, which listed my schedule for the day; to my utter astonishment I saw that Mr. Snellen was scheduled to see me for a consultation at 1:30 PM that afternoon. Michelle and I both looked at each other in amazement, our lower jaws dropping almost to the floor. "Oh, how fate sometime works," I thought. As an internist, I have always lived for diagnostic challenges; cases in medicine in which I get to emulate my hero Mr. Sherlock Holmes. These are the cases in which the clues to the medical mystery might lie in the history given by the patient concerning the particular ailment and its progression, the examination findings, or the former combined with laboratory and x-ray findings. Ninety-five percent of the clues are hidden within the history that the patient narrates to the physician. However, this fact does not absolve the attending physician from doing a thorough examination of the patient as well.

So, it is now 1 PM. I walked into the room and introduced myself to Mr. Snellen and his wife, Margaret. There it was again – the face. But now I had a chance to learn the whole story. I sat down and spent the first ten minutes reviewing the chart that Dr. Martin had developed on Richard and his problems. All of his routine lab work was normal. He had had a chest x-ray and EKG – both of which were within normal limits.

As it turned out, he worked for the city, and every day had to walk up a ramp to the entrance door to his offices. Over the last month he had noted gradually increasing shortness of breath as he made the daily ascending walk up that ramp. At times he had even experienced some chest pain during that climb; he would stop, and the pain would resolve. He had experienced no fever, chills, recent dental work, or obvious infections. He had noted worsening fatigue over the last year, so that just making it through each day had become a real struggle for him. He no longer had any desire for sex; his wife had noted a gradual loss of his hair in the axillary and chest areas. He felt lightheaded at times; but, so far, had not had any fainting spells. Both Richard and his wife told me that Richard had not experienced any trauma to his head, nor had he been hospitalized for any serious illnesses over his lifetime.

My examination of this man was quite informative: His BP when he was lying down was 138/82, but this dropped to 108/68 after I stood him up for two minutes. Since he was not taking any medications that would do this, this drop in pressure is certainly meaningful – occurring with dehydration, pituitary or adrenal gland failure, or a problem with the nerves that help to control a person's blood pressure. The expected findings of hypopituitarism were certainly present: the fine skin and minimal laugh lines; the absence of both axillary and pubic hair; enlarged breasts; and poor muscle mass throughout.   (It is the absence of growth hormone, follicle stimulating hormone, and luteinizing hormone that give rise to the facial findings that I have already described.)   His circulation to his legs was normal. The only unexpected finding that I discovered was a loud murmur emanating from his heart, and which indicated a leak in his mitral valve – the valve that is supposed to shut when the heart contracts, thereby preventing blood from flowing backwards into the patient's lungs. I ordered an EKG, which showed no damage to the heart muscle, but suggested enlargement of his main ventricle; a chest x-ray confirmed the enlargement of Mr. Snellen's heart, together with a small amount of fluid that was now accumulating in his lungs. I saw no masses in either lung.

After Mr. Snellen had dressed, and I had viewed his chest film, I returned to the exam room to discuss my findings and the disorders that I thought were troubling him.

I explained, first of all, that I, indeed, thought that his pituitary gland was not functioning properly; that it was not secreting a number of hormones that tell the other glands in his body to manufacture and secrete their particular hormones. Thus his body was attempting to function, most likely, without the presence of growth hormone, thyroid hormone, the FSH and LH which govern the testicular hormone release, and – most importantly – the cortisol released by the adrenal gland -- a hormone the body needs just to get us through our everyday activities, but which it needs in fairly massive quantities in order to get us through stressful situations such as surgery or a major illness. For example: Our 8 AM morning cortisol level should be 8mcg/dl or slightly higher. If we were to operate on a patient and then measure that cortisol level two hours after the surgery, we should find that it is now around 30mcg/dl – a major increase by the adrenal gland, which, in turn, was all started by the pituitary's increased output of the stimulating hormone ACTH, the hormone governing the adrenal gland's output of cortisol. Without such an increase, the patient could enter an adrenal crisis, with the onset of unrelenting hypotension leading to shock and death.

I explained to both Richard and his wife that there are two hormones that the body absolutely MUST have if it is to maintain life: thyroxine secreted by the thyroid gland and cortisol produced by the adrenal gland. The diminution or absence of the other hormones will certainly make a patient feel bad; but the absence of these two will, ultimately, lead to death. I indicated that I needed to draw blood to check the levels of all of his hormones in order to correctly diagnose his hormone problem. His recent CBC and chemical profile had been normal, with the exception of a mildly decreased sodium level. I explained that – if his cortisol level was borderline – I would then have to do a stimulation test to further evaluate his adrenal function.

In addition, I told them, I was also concerned about his heart – on two levels. On the first level, I was certain that his mitral valve was leaking; and, by allowing fluid to back up into his lungs, that leak was definitely contributing to his shortness of breath as he daily climbed up the ramp to his work. On the second level, the fact that he was experiencing intermittent chest pain with his "ramp exertion" suggested to me that the arteries supplying blood to his heart were narrowed in one or more areas. Therefore, I also needed to investigate his heart -- first by doing an echocardiogram and then with a nuclear stress test. The former would evaluate his overall heart function and also tell me the severity of the leak through the abnormal mitral valve, while the latter test gives evidence of any obstruction which may be present in the arteries that bring blood to the heart muscle.

Both the patient and his wife seemed content with my explanation of his problems and my plan of action. I started Richard on a low dose (20mg) of furosemide every other day in order to remove the fluid from his lungs, and cautioned him to lower his salt intake. Because of the presence of the chest pain, I also had him start low-dose aspirin – 81mg daily. I told him to return the next morning at 8 AM to have all of his hormone levels drawn. I asked Michelle to schedule him for an echocardiogram and a nuclear stress test for Thursday; I would see him back the following week.

I saw Richard back on the Tuesday following his echocardiogram, nuclear stress test, and the drawing of all of his lab values. His lab work did, indeed, confirm the presence of hypopituitarism, with a low cortisol level (3mcg/dl), low ACTH level, an almost undetectable testosterone level (along with decreased FSH and LH Levels), and low thyroid levels with low normal thyroid stimulating hormone numbers. When I reviewed his echocardiogram, I saw that my suspicions were validated: His mitral valve was leaking significantly, but the overall heart function was maintained. However, Richard's nuclear stress test was abnormal, suggesting a possible blockage in the artery that supplies blood to the front wall of the heart – a finding that explained his exertional chest pain and that put him at risk for a major heart attack in the near future.

Richard's case is an excellent example of a patient who presented with multiple problems, which were each, in their own way, contributing to the patient's overall symptom complex. As I taught medical students and residents over my career, I would always remind them that a patient may have "ticks and fleas," meaning that they should always be aware that a patient may have different disease processes that are occurring in parallel with one another. "Occam's Razor" is a concept which tells us that one process should explain all of a patient's symptoms; as physicians, we always consider that possibility first. However, I found that the majority of the patients whom I saw over the years had at least three or more disorders that were attacking their bodies simultaneously.

So, Richard had three major problems present, each in its own way was making him feel totally miserable. Richard and his wife were both shocked by all of this information, but understood the seriousness of his problems.

I first addressed his hypopituitarism, starting him on hydrocortisone 10mg twice a day to replace the cortisol that his adrenal gland was not producing along with low-dose thyroid hormone to begin replacement of that missing hormone. Because of the presence of probable coronary artery disease, I did not put him on testosterone at this time because that hormone might aggravate his cardiac symptoms. Since the pituitary gland was functioning abnormally, I had to be sure that it had not developed a tumor, which was creating the dysfunction; therefore, I had Michelle schedule him for a pituitary-dedicated MRI examination done with contrast. Lastly, I told Richard that he needed to get a medical bracelet which listed his pituitary failure in case he had to go to an ER that was not familiar with him. This bracelet would ensure that his treating physician there would give him adequate amounts of hydrocortisone in order to maintain his blood pressure.

I next discussed with Richard and his wife the cardiac findings. These necessitated a cardiology consultation for further evaluation. He definitely had noticed an improvement in his breathing with the current dose of Furosemide and low-dose aspirin; so I did not change that. I told them that I was referring him to a cardiologist so that he might further evaluate the cardiac problems that I suspected.

Six weeks passed before I saw Richard and his wife back in my office. In the interim he had undergone replacement of his mitral valve as well as coronary artery bypassing of his left anterior descending coronary artery and his right coronary artery – two out of the three vessels supplying the heart with blood and oxygen. He was still a bit fatigued from just having gone through the procedure; but he was improving daily. I had instructed him to double his hydrocortisone dose for the first ten days after the surgery; now he was back on his maintenance dose once again. He was planning on going back to work part time the following week, since he was bored to death just hanging around the house. He was participating in cardiac rehab three times a week, but longed to get back to his job again. He was now on Coumadin (a blood thinner) to prevent a clot from forming on his artificial mitral valve; I now needed to monitor those levels with blood tests every three weeks in order to be sure that the dose of that drug was correct. If his level wasn't high enough, then he might form a blood clot on the valve, which could then break off and travel to his brain, thus causing a stroke. If the level were to become too high, he would then have a much higher risk of bleeding -- usually from the stomach or intestine.

At the time of his next visit a month later Richard was feeling good. He was now working full time, and no longer suffered the chest pain and shortness of breath that plagued him earlier. He had decided to continue the cardiac rehab for maintenance of his physical strength. This he continued even up to the time of my retirement in March, 2015. During the years following his valve replacement, Richard had one bleeding episode, which, at endoscopy, was seen to originate from a colonic polyp, which the gastroenterologist removed.

And so, in this case, as in others that smolder for a time, the patient's symptoms very gradually developed: first the libido and sexual dysfunction became a problem; then fatigue developed, followed by the cardiac symptoms – with both hypopituitarism and his heart problems ultimately combining, making Richard miserable. Richard's facial features provided the initial clue that allowed me to make the diagnosis of hypopituitarism, a life-threatening condition; while the physical exam not only confirmed that diagnosis it also identified one of the two other heart problems that had to be addressed. These were surgically corrected, so that he no longer suffered exertional chest pain or shortness of breath. However, we had now committed him to a lifetime of blood thinner therapy in order to prevent clots from developing on the artificial heart valve, which could then break loose and travel (most often) to the brain, producing an embolic stroke and paralysis. One can see that the obvious side effect of such therapy is bleeding, which most often occurs from a source in the gastrointestinal tract – such as an ulcer, gastritis, diverticulosis, or a tumor in any part of the tract. A fall with a minor degree of head trauma can give rise to a bleed into the brain – which often is fatal. Warfarin is the only blood-thinner that is still currently approved for use in treating patients with artificial valves in place, and treatment with this drug necessitates frequent blood testing in order to adjust the dosage. We now have three other anticoagulants available, which act on a specific part of the coagulation system; so that they are safer and require no blood monitoring (except for checking a blood count occasionally to look for anemia). Research is ongoing to see if we might one day use the newer drugs in heart-valve patients, thus making Warfarin a medical dinosaur. I can only hope, both for the patients' and the doctors' sakes, that this might happen soon.

Once again, I – along with his cardiologist – followed Richard in our office until I retired in March of 2015. He continued to do well, with occasional readjustment of some of his heart medications. He certainly represents, along with some of the other patients whom I have already discussed, one of the most interesting and complex patients I saw while in Sweetwater; and it had all begun with a fleeting glance at his face while in the hallway that day.

CHAPTER 8

PEGGY HANSEN

Many changes occurred in medicine with the passage of the Affordable Care Act in 2010. –. Some of these changes were for the better: for example, the greedy insurance people could no longer exclude people who had "pre-existing" conditions from coverage, nor could they price them out the insurance market entirely by merely establishing exorbitant premiums for those types of patients. Considering that a fifty year-old man or woman coming into my office most often has at least five or six disorders (hypertension, diabetes, hyperlipidemia, osteoarthritis, etc.), this provision of the act was an extremely important step in allowing these patients affordable access to continued medical care, especially as they aged and became afflicted with even more medical problems with which we physicians had to deal.

The Affordable Care Act also provided funds so that states could expand Medicaid, which would now give poorer people access to medical care – a benefit that they had lacked for years. Many states took advantage of this funding, while others chose not to do so; with their citizens and hospitals suffering because of that choice.

However, the Affordable Care Act introduced another feature to the practice of medicine, which has forever changed its nature; and not for the better. This was the requirement that the Electronic Health Record now be utilized to document the care that a physician provides to his patients. This "innovation" was touted by the government to be a means by which the quality of health care delivery would be improved. No longer would a physician be allowed to dictate into the medical record the patient's history, the physical examination, along with the assessment and plan for that patient's care – no matter how complicated the problems of that patient might be. Instead, the bean counters demanded that we try to document all of these things by clicking boxes that have symptoms and/or simple physical findings associated with them. This process makes it much easier for those counters to analyze the medical record for payment purposes – even though that record may, in no manner, explain what is really going on with the patient.

For example, if I were to admit a patient to the ICU who was in a coma my dictation on that patient would need to contain information concerning how the episode had begun, my findings on the general physical examination of the patient, along with documentation of the detailed neurologic examination of that person. My narrative would also need to include details concerning laboratory and imaging data (such as a CT scan of the head); so that, at the end of the dictation, I might formulate diagnoses and plans for management of this unfortunate individual. Therefore, my dictation concerning this patient would be at least three to four pages long. The EHR at our hospital had only six boxes that I might "click" concerning a neurological exam of a patient whom I might admit to the hospital – none of which applied to a patient such as I have just discussed.

I AM sure that all of you have noticed over the last few years that your physician spends ninety-five percent of your visit time with him typing or "clicking" boxes on his computer. He or she might listen to your heart for ten seconds and, perhaps listen to your lungs; however, that is probably the extent of the examination no matter what problems you are dealing with. It is rare in this day and age that a physician might ask a patient to disrobe a certain area of the body so that he or she might perform a complete examination of the area. I was recently admitted to the hospital with severe abdominal pain brought on by acute diverticulitis. The "internist-hospitalist" spent a total of ten minutes with me on admission; her physical examination consisted in a handshake, a ten-second listen to my heart, and a brief auscultation of my lungs. She never examined my abdomen – which was the reason for my admission – nor any other part of my body. Yet I AM certain that she "clicked" all of the little boxes that briefly and inadequately described my condition. Indeed, she never examined my abdomen during the three days of my stay in that hospital. I was still having abdominal pain when she discharged me on oral antibiotics after three days on IV antibiotics. Fortunately, I had an appointment to see a gastroenterologist three days later. He actually obtained a history from me; and, after examining my abdomen and reviewing the CT scan, promptly admitted me for six days to a different hospital for IV antibiotic treatment of my unresolved acute diverticulitis. The "hospitalist" at the second hospital certainly performed better than the person at the first hospital, but still not at a level that I would expect from the medicine residents whom I had mentored over my career.

And so the Affordable Care Act basically dispensed with true and accurate medical care, replacing it with a "board game," in which the one who has the most "clicks" gets paid more than those who have less boxes checked. With this system, hospitals (especially rural hospitals) suffer significant loss in reimbursement if the attending physicians don't understand how to play the game well. There are two losers in this process. First of all, we the patients lose because the physician, anchored to the EHR, is denied time to perform an accurate history and physical exam on us – unless he or she is willing to see fewer patients daily and thereby expect less pay. Secondly, the hospital gets less reimbursement should their physicians not be taught how to play the "game" correctly. As long as the government demands the use of the electronic health record, good medical care to the individual patient will be lost forever; for without an accurate history and examination, diagnoses WILL be missed. I retired in March, 2015. Even up until that time I refused to do other than dictate all of my notes – both in the office and at the hospital. I knew that I would soon be penalized by CMS (Medicare) for continuing this practice (or, perhaps, be fired by my clinic.); so that these facts, along with some health issues, led me to my decision to retire.

However, around November, 2014 Peggy Hansen arrived at our Rolling Plains Memorial Hospital. Peggy had been a nurse and nurse practitioner for many years, and had worked in administrative positions as well. Having recognized early on the "board game" nature of the EHR; but, at the same time knowing how important it was that hospitals and physicians be reimbursed correctly for all of the care that they give to very complicated patients, she now was working as a consultant, traveling to hospitals all over the country in order to teach their physicians how to document in the EHR thoroughly enough that the everyone involved in the care of these very sick patients would be paid for the care they were rendering to them.

Peggy was grounded in the nursing care itself, in administrative processes, and – even more importantly – in the coding process now utilized by Medicare and other insurances for reimbursement purposes. All of us at the hospital soon realized how smart Peggy was. Her knowledge of her subject was encyclopedic. Furthermore, the wit and enthusiasm that she demonstrated in teaching made the entire process a true learning experience for all of us. The knowledge that she imparted to us physicians during her week at our small hospital has allowed it to thrive and be reimbursed as it should be.

After Peggy and I had finished reviewing some of my hospital charts one afternoon, she told me something that surprised me. She said, "I have been to hospitals all over the country reviewing medical records, and I have never seen notes as good as yours. As I read them I find myself able to follow your patients' progress, along with your thought processes, almost as if I were reading a novel about them. After you retire might you be interested in writing a book about the extraordinary cases that you have seen in your practice of rural medicine? I told Peggy that I would think about that.

I retired, and my wife, Alicia, and I moved back to her home town of San Antonio in April, 2015. Peggy and I kept in touch; later Peggy, her husband Jim Aucoin, Alicia, and I all met for dinner in San

Antonio. At that time, both she and Jim indicated that they were interested in my book. Jim gave me some titles of a couple of books that he thought I should read before beginning to write my own; these I read over the next two months. I then began my own narrative.

CHAPTER 9

THE HEART OF THE MATTER

W hen Peggy Hansen asked me to write this book, she was most interested that I discuss the more unusual diseases and disorders that occurred rarely in medicine. The fact that I was able to make these diagnoses while practicing in an area far distant from cities with their many specialists fascinated her; she was very interested in alerting the public to what a thorough practice of medicine could accomplish – and that one did not need a "total body CT scanner" in order to make an accurate diagnosis in a patient. Many of the diagnoses that I have discussed up to this point I suspected or even made during my taking of a detailed history from the patient, with the laboratory and/or imaging studies merely confirming that which I already knew was afflicting that person. One diagnosis evidenced itself merely from my inspection of the patient's facial features in the hallway. I admit that I sometimes had to spend thirty-five to forty-five minutes interviewing the patient in order to be certain that I had heard his or her story correctly, while during other encounters I might need only ten to fifteen minutes in order to obtain adequate historical information from the patient.

The disorder that I now will discuss is exceedingly rare (with an incidence of 0.0017 and 0.19% of unselected autopsies.). That is definitely a rare disease.

This rarity truly smolders within its victim for years before it begins to manifest its presence; it does so ever so subtly, making it one of the great "mimics" that we occasionally come across in medicine. One such "mimic' is acute appendicitis, which may present with symptoms that suggest other intra-abdominal conditions in a patient with abdominal pain, depending on the position of the appendix within that patient's abdomen. Syphilis, with its three stages, mimics many other disorders as it progresses through those stages (each one manifesting different symptoms); so that it, like acute appendicitis, can easily be misdiagnosed. Endocarditis, which usually involves an infection of a heart valve, can mimic rheumatoid arthritis in its early stages. The extremely rare problem that I encountered one cold January evening in 2010, had truly proven itself over the years to fall into this category. A patient with this disease might present with minor symptoms of arthritis or arthritis symptoms so bad that his physician (and even the rheumatologist) suspects that he or she has rheumatoid arthritis. The poor victim of this process might present with prolonged fevers suggesting an infection somewhere. On the other hand, the patient might present with a stroke, fainting spells, kidney failure, or heart failure – truly proving it to be a chameleon with its various presentations.

Now, I really hate being cold. If the temperature drops to eighty degrees, I would be perfectly happy if I might find a nice warm rock on which I could recline. The temperature on this late January afternoon was a balmy 28 degrees. My nurse watched and chuckled as I put on my multiple layers of clothing along with my ski hat in order to traverse the distance between our clinic and the hospital across the street (total distance being about the length of two football fields.). It had snowed a couple of days before; but that snow had now turned to ice – making the journey that I was about to commence somewhat dangerous for a man of sixty-seven years afflicted with significant osteoporosis.

I slowly inched my way through our parking lot and then onto the street. Some of the ice on the street had melted, making my trek through that area safer. I just had to negotiate the slight hill leading to the front door of the hospital, and I'd be home free. Again, using the "inching technique," I managed to complete this final leg of my trip, and entered the safety of the foyer of the hospital. During each winter that I was in Sweetwater I always felt relief when I finally opened that front door of the hospital at the end of these adventures.

I walked to the medical-surgical floor, shed my layers of winter clothing, and obtained the patient's current medical record along with her old hospital charts. I settled into a chair in the physicians' dictation room, and began my review of her records.

I had been asked by a local surgeon to see this patient. He basically was asking me to "clear" this patient for a proposed gallbladder resection that he had planned for the next morning.

Such a request for an internist to consult on a patient is fairly common, with the request usually coming from a general surgeon or orthopedic specialist. Often the proposed surgical patient has multiple medical problems that the specialist wants evaluated before the patient enters the operating room.

The surgeon's current history and physical seemed to indicate that this sixty-nine- year-old female patient had been experiencing abdominal bloating, occasional nausea, and some pain high in the right upper quadrant for a number of months. She had hypertension for a number of years, which had been poorly controlled.

She had smoked two packs of cigarettes daily for at least ten years. Routine laboratory studies showed no evidence for anemia, diabetes, or kidney problems. Her sonogram report demonstrated some stones in her gallbladder. For these reasons, the surgeon felt that a cholecystectomy was indicated. The EKG and chest x-ray reports were normal.

There were two old charts from previous admissions available for my review. The first record concerned itself with an emergency room visit for minor trauma to her leg four years before this admission; it contained no useful data that would help with her current problem.

Her other record, however, proved to be more informative. The lady had been admitted to our hospital one-and-one-half years ago with fever, chills, and joint pains. Her blood cultures were negative for any organism growth, while the urine grew an E.coli bug – a common cause of urinary infections in women. Her chest x-ray was read as normal, thus ruling out the presence of pneumonia. While her liver and kidney functions were normal, her CBC showed a slight elevation of her white blood cell count – consistent with her infection. I was just about to close the chart, when I noticed another blood test at the bottom of the CBC report.

Her attending physician had done another blood test during that admission that did not just merely "catch my eye," but made me look at this patient in an entirely different light – a test result that gave me my first clue that this case was about a patient afflicted by much more than a simple gallbladder problem. "God bless old hospital charts," I said to myself as I stared at the result of the sedimentation rate test ordered by her physician during that admission; for the reported result was 127 millimeters/hour.

Aside from doing a simple urinalysis, this particular blood test is about as simple a test that exists in medicine: one simply draws blood from a patient, puts it into a tube, and observes the rate at which the red blood cells settle out. The test is a gross measure of any inflammation that may be present in a person; for, in the presence of an inflammatory process, the patient's body releases proteins into the bloodstream, which cover the red blood cells and make them heavier than they usually are. These cells then settle to the bottom of the tube more quickly. The red cells normally will move toward the bottom of the tube at a rate of 20 millimeters/hour – a normal result. As we age, normal results rise slightly up to about 30 millimeters/hour. I was staring at a sedimentation rate of 127 mm/hour. This result was not compatible with a simple urinary tract infection; rather, this level suggested that this patient had a major inflammatory disease process ongoing at the time of that hospitalization that had not yet been diagnosed. There are only a small number of diseases that will raise a sedimentation rate to levels greater than 100mm/hour. So, as I walked to the patient's room to begin my consultation, I knew that the odds of my making a correct diagnosis in this patient had just risen significantly.

I entered her room and introduced myself; she had been expecting me. I pulled a chair close to the bed, sat down, and asked her to tell me her story – starting from the very beginning of her symptoms. The subject was about five feet eight inches tall, with brown eyes and grey hair. She looked to be older than her stated age, with deep wrinkles on her face along with multiple actinic keratosis – both of which suggested long term exposure to cigarette smoke and to sunlight. She continued to lie in bed as she narrated her story to me.

Sarah told me that she had felt good until about two years ago, when she noticed occasional stiffness and soreness in her hands, which were accompanied by a feeling of a lack of energy. She told me that her last admission was precipitated by the advent of fever, chills, joint pains, and burning with urination. No other symptoms manifested until about July of last year, when she began to experience some shortness of breath when she would make the bed or vacuum the rugs. She told me that her blood pressure had been poorly controlled; but that she had no history of diabetes, kidney disease, swelling in her legs, heart murmur, nor any cough or chest pain. Sarah denied any street drug use. She had never been anemic, and she gave me no history of any skin problems. She indicated that, over the last two months, her shortness of breath had worsened. In addition, she had noticed a feeling of fullness when she ate, along with mild nausea – both of which were easily relieved with Tums. At no time had she suffered severe right upper abdominal pain, fevers, chills, vomiting, or evidence for jaundice. I was beginning to wonder if I was talking with the person who had been described in the current medical chart; for, so far, I had not elicited symptoms that suggested significant gallbladder disease. I finally finished taking her history, and began my examination of Sarah.

Her routine vital signs, including oxygen levels, were normal. Examination of her upper and lower extremities revealed completely normal findings, except for those skin findings upon which I commented earlier. I found no abnormal finding on examination of her head and neck, nor any tenderness on feeling the arteries that ran along each side of her head; a search for enlarged lymph glands revealed none.

I now turned my attention to her abdomen. It was not distended, and I noted a healed appendectomy scar in the right lower quadrant. She had no abdominal pain when I shook her abdomen and none as I gently percussed the entire area. I now began to deeply palpate her abdomen, and found no masses or tenderness – even in the gallbladder region. Her liver and spleen were also normal. My testing of a stool sample obtained when I did the rectal exam revealed no evidence for blood loss from anywhere in her GI tract.

After I completed her lung exam (which was normal), I ended my interrogation of her body by conducting a complete cardiac examination, part of which involves listening to her heart sounds while I have Sarah in different positions – while she is on her back, with her sitting on the edge of the bed and leaning forward, and while she lay in bed on her left side. In her case the cardiac exam remained normal until I listened to her heart while she was on her side. With her in that position I heard a very distinct "swooshing" sound that is characteristic of a heart murmur; in this case the murmur indicated that the heart's mitral valve was leaking – thereby allowing blood to go backward from her left ventricle (chamber) into her lung. However, just at the end of that murmur I heard another sound that was totally unfamiliar to me; it was a very brief and dull "thump." I listened to her heart in all positions once again; but it was only when Sarah lay on her left side that I heard both of the sounds. After I had completed my exam, I left the room to review her x-rays, EKG tracing, and the abdominal sonogram.

Her EKG tracing definitely had subtle findings that suggested enlargement of her left atrium – the chamber through which blood flows from the lungs into the main pumping chamber of the heart. I found her chest x-ray to be normal; however, so was her abdominal sonogram. The gallbladder was not enlarged nor did it contain any stones. Its walls were of normal thickness and there was no fluid around the organ -- both findings indicating a LACK of any gallbladder inflammation.

After I completed all of these activities, I was absolutely convinced that Sarah had no gallbladder problems whatsoever, and that she certainly did not need a cholecystectomy. I felt, however, that she was suffering from an ongoing systemic inflammatory process that was evidenced during her hospital stay one-and-one-half years ago by the grossly elevated sedimentation rate of 127mm/hour. So I called the attending surgeon and discussed this patient's problems with him – indicating that I felt that he should certainly not proceed with his proposed surgery to remove her gallbladder. He was unhappy to hear this recommendation, but was slightly less peeved when I further explained to him the reason for my decision; the scheduled surgery was cancelled.

I mentioned earlier that my odds of making a correct diagnosis had gone up considerably after seeing such a markedly elevated sedimentation rate; for there are a limited number of diseases that will produce that much inflammation in a patient's body. My odds got even better after my very careful examination of her heart -- especially after hearing that murmur along with the other abnormal sound. Her heart, in my mind, was most likely the culprit, giving rise to both her symptoms and the lab findings. And that extra sound ... could it be?

I repeated her sedimentation rate, and drew blood cultures to be sure that she did not have endocarditis, which is an infection of the heart valves. (That infection is also one of the great mimics in medicine.) I checked for all of the "collagen-vascular" diseases with the appropriate blood tests – these include rheumatoid arthritis, lupus and its variants, and diseases known as "vasculitis," in which the body attacks its own blood vessels. Multiple myeloma (a cancer originating from one of our infection-fighting cells) can also raise the sedimentation rate this high; so I had the lab draw the protein studies to check for this. An occult malignancy (especially lymphoma) is another culprit that can produce this kind of result. However, I had found no enlarged lymph nodes on exam, and there were no tumor or enlarged nodes visible on her chest x-ray or sonogram. Sarah had had a normal colonoscopy about a year ago; I found her breast exam to be normal.

I was beginning to think that Sarah had a disorder that I might see only once in my lifetime – an atrial myxoma. This is a tumor that arises from the inner lining of the heart. It contains many different kinds of heart cells, from early primordial cells all the way to fully differentiated inner cardiac lining cells. As it grows, the tumor projects into the cardiac chamber of origin, which is almost always the left atrium. Most resemble a polyp and are often on a stalk, which makes them mobile within the chamber. Because of this mobility, they can interfere with closure of a cardiac valve, which is what I thought was occurring in Sarah.

These tumors may cause the patient to have generalized symptoms, thus mimicking all of the disorders that I have mentioned. The precise mechanism by which this happens is unclear. Because a myxoma is an abnormal structure inside of the heart, in thirty-forty percent of cases blood clots may form on them, which can then travel in the blood stream to the brain or any other organ, causing devastating consequences. The mobility of these tumors may prevent the mitral valve (most often) from closing, or – worse yet – it may "plop" into the opening of the valve area and cause sudden death. So, not only can a myxoma in a patient be a fantastic mimic of other generalized disorders, but also, because of its position in the heart, it can cause heart failure, embolism, intra cardiac infections, and even sudden cardiac death. I ordered her echocardiogram at the same time that I ordered all of the other blood tests; for in this report should lie the answer to the mystery.

Once again, her sedimentation rate was elevated above 100mm/hour. All of the other tests were negative for the diseases for which I was testing. On the day following my consultation Sarah had her echocardiogram performed; and there it was. The tumor was about an inch in diameter and anchored on a stalk to the septum that divides the left from the right atria. With contraction of the left atrium it would descend and prevent the back leaflet of the mitral valve from closing – thereby causing that valve to leak. This mechanism (along with the tumor mass) contributed to Sarah's shortness of breath. However, the echo also showed that her left ventricle had become fairly "stiff" and noncompliant because of her years of poorly controlled hypertension; this fact also would contribute to her breathing difficulty. The presence of the tumor also explained the fatigue and arthritis symptoms that she'd been having over the past two years.

I thought back to the beginning of this journey when the results of one of the simplest lab tests in the world had, ultimately, started me on the road to this diagnosis, and I again thanked the "Medical Record Gods" for their favor granted.

I explained to Sarah and her husband, James, in great detail the nature of the diagnosis along with the fact that this tumor would definitely have to be removed, for it could grow fairly rapidly. Thereafter, I spoke with my cardiologist in Abilene, and arranged a transfer so that he could complete the rest of the diagnostic evaluation necessary prior to surgery.

As it turned out, because of the extreme rarity of this problem, the cardiovascular surgeons in Abilene felt uncomfortable doing the operation. They referred her to cardiac surgeons in Dallas, who were able to remove the tumor without having to replace Sarah's mitral valve.

I saw Sarah back in a month and she was doing much better. She had no arthritis symptoms and her fatigue had improved. Although her shortness of breath had improved, she still noticed it whenever she tried to exert herself a bit more than usual. She continued the two-pack per day smoking. Her sedimentation rate was now only 32mm/hour.

I followed Sarah until I retired. She developed diastolic heart failure because of the "stiffness" of her heart muscle, the latter resulting from the years of hypertension. I was able to control both the hypertension and the heart failure with medical treatment; the cardiologist saw her every six months. Repeat echocardiograms failed to show any recurrence of her tumor over a five-year period. Unfortunately she never did stop smoking and developed emphysema severe enough to require treatment with oxygen during the last two years that I cared for her.

Sarah's atrial myxoma is truly the rarest of all of the somewhat rare conditions that I diagnosed while I practiced in Sweetwater – or in any of my practice locations. Yet I was able to suspect the diagnosis, not because I had a "total-body CT scanner" at my disposal, but because I took the time to review records and to perform a true cardiac examination on this woman. If I had not listened to her heart while she lay on her left side, I would have missed the final clue that led me to the correct diagnosis. Good physical examination led to this rare diagnosis – Hamilton Bailey and Sherlock should be proud.

CHAPTER 10

A MISSED OPPORTUNITY

S weetwater resembles a lot of the towns in rural Texas. There are usually two or three industries in the towns that support employment, thereby helping to keep people living there; the two gypsum mills and our hospital were the main employers. Multiple burger joints, barbecue restaurants, and fried chicken eateries comprised the local cuisine. Unfortunately, not all of the rural towns were fortunate enough to have a local hospital, especially with the changes that have occurred in medicine over the past few years. We were lucky to have a "hospital district," so that a portion of the property taxes collected from the residents went toward maintenance of the hospital.

The Rolling Plains Memorial Hospital where I admitted patients for care is an excellent facility. It has fifty-four beds that include a five-bed ICU, a medical-surgical ward, and a smaller section devoted to obstetrics. The nurses who staffed the hospital were superb; they had a good knowledge of nursing care along with an abundance of common sense. If any one of them called me about a patient who they felt was not doing well, I knew that I needed to get to the hospital to assess the patient as soon as possible. (These talented and caring persons cared for me during my five admissions to the hospital over my time in Sweetwater – all of which were for very serious illnesses. I was certainly in good hands.) The hospital had

CT scanning capabilities; later a mobile MRI scanner became a permanent fixture, making our diagnostic capabilities even better.

I have heard people say over the years that good medical care can only be obtained in a big city hospital, and certainly not in a small town facility such as ours. Oh, how wrong those people are. (My own experiences in the hospitals of San Antonio have certainly confirmed the fallacy of that argument. During my many admissions since arriving here in April, 2015, I wished many times that I were back in the Rolling Plains hospital.) We could care well for many patients with critical illnesses in our facility, but would ship any patient having a heart attack immediately to a cardiologist in Abilene. Although not formally trained in critical care, I was forced to obtain these skills early on during my practice in Rupert, Idaho, as we had to deal with critical patients in our twenty-five bed hospital; I studied the critical care articles in the *New England Journal of Medicine*, and read the critical care textbooks by both James Rippe and Jesse Hall during my career. So, along with the great ICU nursing staff, I managed all of the very critically ill patients at the request of my family practice colleagues. One of the surgeons on staff was excellent and performed major operations meticulously and with great skill. When my colon perforated in December, 2007, he explored my abdomen, removed part of my colon, and created my colostomy for me – obviously a major operation. He left for another position around 2010, but we were lucky to have a female surgeon, Summer Waltham, join the staff shortly thereafter who was equally skilled in her profession; so I referred all of my surgical patients to her until I left in 2015.

Late one afternoon in October, 2009, June, who worked in the pre-op area of the hospital, entered my office and asked to speak with me. Now, my office was always cluttered. But there was a small chair directly in front of my desk; so she managed to slither into that and began to tell the tale of her father, whom she wanted me to see.

Her father, Jim, was in his late sixties, living in Snyder, about a thirty-minute drive from Sweetwater. He began to suffer symptoms that suggested a sinus infection in July. A physician saw him, and treated him with appropriate antibiotics. However, his symptoms recurred once again while he was in Brownwood, Texas, a month later. Treated again by a local physician for both infection and allergies, he seemed to improve a bit; however, he still experienced some mild nasal drainage. His symptoms recurred in September – and now he was beginning to feel worse, with headache, severe fatigue, and occasional nosebleeds. His local physician again treated Jim with antibiotics – but Jim demonstrated no improvement. As late September approached, he noticed persistent nasal drainage, increasing weakness, and had now developed a cough that was associated with shortness of breath. At the time of my conversation with June, Jim could barely move around at all.

I questioned June about any other symptoms that her father may have had; these included a low grade fever, but he had experienced no gastrointestinal problems, and he had developed no rashes. He did mention that his joints were slightly painful over the past two months. June mentioned that her father's urine output had decreased over the past three days.

As I listened to June narrate her father's story, I realized what disease was mounting this vicious attack on her father and that he was now in very critical condition because of its effects on his lungs and kidneys. I told her to bring him as a direct admission to the ICU of our hospital, and to have the nurses call me when he arrived.

It is our body's ability to mount an "inflammatory response" that is such an important reason that we are able to live as long as we do. If one of us, for example, were to develop an attack of acute appendicitis, the body mobilizes white blood cells of different types to the infected region, which then triggers the release of a series of proteins known as "complement." Together, these generate inflammation in order to limit this potentially malicious infection to a small area of our body. This allows the physician both to diagnose the problem at an early stage and to cure the disorder by prompt removal of the infected and inflamed appendix.

However, these same inflammatory processes, which usually help to defend us from infections, may actually cause many diseases –

diseases may be slowly progressive, such as rheumatoid arthritis and other arthritis states like ankylosing spondylitis, an arthritis affecting the joints of the lower back and the spine. These diseases fall into the "autoimmune disease" category, in which the inflammatory process seems to be aimed at antigens that did not come from some infective organism, but are antigens that are inherent in our own bodies.

Unfortunately, within this group of autoimmune diseases there are disorders that cause inflammation within the walls of blood vessels in our body, which makes the lumen of the involved vessel much smaller than normal. When the pathologist reviews the biopsy of an affected vessel he or she will visualize inflammatory white cells and proteins within the walls of the vessels, with that inflammation creating a narrowing of the lumen of those affected blood vessels One can induce from the fact of this narrowing that the organ supplied with blood by this artery will now lack that precious oxygen-laden liquid, and will eventually lose its ability to function. The disease giving rise to such vascular inflammation is called a "vasculitis," of which there are many types -- classified based on the size of the blood vessel that is the victim of their attack.

For example, "giant cell arteritis" is a vasculitis that inflames the large vessels such as the aorta, vessels supplying blood to the stomach and intestines, and even the arteries that bring blood to the brain. This disease may cause the patient to complain of headaches, abdominal pain, or even unilateral blindness. The patient usually feels tired, is anemic, and often complains of shoulder pain.

As June told me her father's story, I became convinced that he was suffering from a small vessel vasculitis known as "granulomatosis with polyangiitis" (formerly known as "Wegener's granulomatosis), a name which gave credit to one of its discoverers. The disorder can attack any organ, but its main pattern of involvement involves inflammation in the vessels in the nose and sinuses, the lung (where it not only causes inflammation, but also may produce diffuse lung hemorrhage from rupture of the smallest vessels), the skin, muscles and nerves, and the kidneys; here it produces nephritis and progressive kidney failure.

The patient with this vasculitis will most often present to his physician with symptoms resembling a sinus infection, just as Jim had initially done. Unfortunately, his treating physicians had never recognized that these symptoms truly represented the early embers of this somewhat rare disorder, even after their evaluation of Jim on many occasions. It is because of the existence of these vasculitis disorders that I always taught my residents and medical students to order a sedimentation rate on patients whose sinus problems were persisting; the results in these disorders, which usually return at levels greater than 100mm/hour in almost all cases, gives the attending physician a major clue to presence of such inflammation.

Around seven-thirty Shauna called from ICU to notify me of Jim's arrival, and indicated that he certainly did not look good. I was still at my office, so I told her to order blood cultures, a CBC, CMP (which evaluates electrolytes, glucose levels, and both kidney and liver function), and a sedimentation rate. I told her that we also needed a urinalysis, serum lactic acid level, measurement of an arterial blood gas, chest x-ray, EKG, and cardiac enzymes drawn – therefore, when I arrived at the hospital, I would have data available for analysis on this man with multisystem disease. The last test that I ordered is a test that is a serum marker for the specific disease that I suspected in this patient -- an ANCA panel. This test detects antibodies that specifically react with the antigens in cytoplasmic granules within the white blood cell. First discovered by Dr. DJ Davis and his associates in 1982, this test has now proven itself to be present in up to ninety percent of patients with small-vessel vasculitis.

I entered the ICU around 8 PM. Our ICU was arranged in such a way that, as one comes through the door the large, semicircular nursing station is just to the right. The nurses have a two-tier desk, with the monitors on the top level and their computers on the lower level. From this vantage point they are able to see all five of the ICU beds. Just behind the nursing station there is a desk with a computer on which the physicians could enter their orders (and "click" the history and physical, if the physician chose that route). Also on the desk is a large monitor, on which one could visualize the order input, nursing notes, lab data, and also view x-rays which had been done on the patients. By now the lab had drawn all of the blood specimens, and Shauna had attached the heart monitor and placed an IV so that we would have access to his veins. Since he was not able to pass any urine, I had ordered that a bladder catheter be placed as well. Radiology had just finished taking his portable chest x-ray. There was no data for me to review at this point; so I entered the first ICU bed room to begin my evaluation of Jim Simmons.

Jim certainly looked to be ill; weight loss was obvious in the loss of muscle mass in his facial muscles and in the muscles of his arms. Because of his generalized weakness, he had great difficulty in trying to change positions in the bed. He stated his age to be sixty-nine; however, he appeared to be much older than that.

I pulled a chair next to the bedside and took his history; it was essentially the same story that June had already told me. Of great concern to me was his development of a cough along with the worsening shortness of breath over the last week to ten days along with the fact that he had passed no urine over the past two days. I now began my exam.

Jim's blood pressure was 140/74, with a pulse rate of 88. His oxygen saturation while on room air was only 83% (normal being greater than 95%). After taking that measurement, Shauna had already started him on oxygen. His level was now 92%; however, he was breathing at a rate of thirty breaths per minute in order to maintain his level in that range. Examination of his head and neck region revealed the ravages of his disease process; the lining of his nasal passages looked as if some creature had been nibbling on it, for there were small pieces of the mucosa (lining) that were missing, while the remainder of the mucosa was completely irritated with areas of slight bleeding visible. I found his ears, mouth and neck to be normal. I detected pallor in the upper and lower eyelids, suggesting the presence of an anemia.

I next examined his heart, abdomen and skin, and found them all to be normal. However, upon listening to his lungs, I heard abnormal sounds throughout both of them – sounds that could signify fluid or inflammation throughout his lung tissue, abnormalities that would explain his shortness of breath and low oxygen level.

By now most of Jim's lab work had returned, most of which was abnormal. His CBC proved the existence of an anemia, with an hemoglobin of 8.5g/dl and a hematocrit of 28%. The white blood count was elevated at 22,000, while the platelet count (small particles in the blood which help to stop a person from bleeding) was only 52,000 (normal being greater than 150,000).

But it was the CMP, arterial blood gas report, and chest x-ray which truly got my attention. These results indicated that Jim's kidneys had stopped working and that he was now in full-blown acute kidney failure. The CMP revealed a BUN of 95mg/dl and a creatinine level of 6.8 mg/dl -- kidney tests which normally measure a BUN of less than 20mg/dl and a creatinine of around 1.3mg/dl. His bicarbonate level was low, which indicated that the renal failure had allowed the accumulation of excess acids in his system, a fact that was also confirmed by his arterial gas measurement demonstrating a pH of 7.2 (normal being 7.4).

I considered all of these findings to be very worrisome; however, after looking at Jim's chest x-ray and the rest of his blood gas report, I realized that his granulomatous disease had now advanced so far as to produce both kidney and lung failure -- the end stage of this aggressive process. The remainder of his blood gas report revealed that not only could this man not maintain his oxygen level adequately, his lungs, which were filled up with inflammation, were now becoming unable to get rid of the carbon dioxide from his body – as manifested by an elevated PCO_2 level of 64 (normal is 24). His sedimentation rate value returned at greater than 150mm/hour

There was little that I could do for this poor man at this point. I started him on antibiotics to treat any infection and high dose solu-medrol to begin to treat his disease. I called my pulmonary specialist in Abilene, explaining to her the problem that I thought my patient had as well as the dire straits in which I now found him. I now needed to transfer him to her for further care of this rare problem, which was nearly at its end stage. After she agreed, I had the anesthetist intubate Jim, so that I could put him on the ventilator and breath for him; we had to have control of his airway and breathing from here on out. Fifteen minutes later, the ambulance crew arrived for the transfer, taking Mr. Simmons to the ICU at Abilene Regional Medical Center.

A couple of days went by, and then I received a call from the consultant during which she told me that Jim had expired. Although she had added Cyclophosphamide (the second drug used to treat this disease), his lungs had worsened; when she scoped those lungs, she found diffuse bleeding throughout. He did not have a bacterial pneumonia nor bugs growing in his blood. The PR3-ANCA level was grossly elevated, though, thus helping to confirm the diagnosis of granulomatosis with polyangiitis.

A number of different physicians had an encounter with this patient, yet they failed to make the correct diagnosis at a time when early treatment of this disease would have allowed him possibly to even be alive today. Granted, the embers of this process were very tiny at first; but, oh how they grew and spread! This is surely a case about which Sherlock would comment, "If you are unaware of the existence of something, then you won't know to look for it." If a physician is not familiar with medicine's rarer cases– has not read enough about the "Zebra" patient who occasionally walks into his or her exam room – then the correct diagnosis will leave that physician's office as the patient walks out of the front door. Unfortunately, some of these rarer diseases are very deadly in their progression. As I thought about this case over the years, I always wished that I had seen Jim in July, when there was a chance to put him in remission.

CHAPTER 11

AN EXCRUCIATING PAIN

So disease embers can smolder but gradually spread and enlarge to the point where a knowledgeable physician will recognize the process for what it is; that it is an illness, which, if left unchecked, will ultimately disable or even kill the affected patient. However, other disorders (such as the anaphylaxis which I discussed much earlier) are not of that ilk. Rather, they start suddenly and with viciousness so intense that the illness disables the patient immediately. Furthermore, some of these conflagrations prove exceedingly difficult to control. The mystery here consists not in the disease diagnosis, but, rather how the physician (most often with specialist help) is going to control the disorder to the point where that patient functions again and lives a normal life. And so I now come to a discussion of such a process, a discussion of a disease that can generate so much pain that, before there was any form of treatment for the excruciating pain that it produces, the most common cause of death in these unfortunate people was suicide.

Lori Bender had worked in administration at Rolling Plains Memorial Hospital for a few years before I arrived in September, 2000. I would pass her office daily on my way to see patients in the ICU. Often I would stop to talk with her for a few minutes to see how she and her family were doing. Sometimes she would run out to catch me in the hallway saying, "Dr. Kassis, Dr. Kassis, I have a good joke for you." Then she would either tell me her joke or show me the cartoon that illustrated it.

At this time Lori was in her middle thirties, tall (5 feet, ten inches), with brown hair that fell to just below her ears. She possessed an infectious laugh; everyone who worked with her immediately became her friend. Life was truly going well for Lori; she had a loving husband, Mike, great kids, and a good job. However, all of this was to change dramatically one Thursday afternoon in 2003.

Lori was working at her desk that Thursday afternoon in August, when her cohorts heard her suddenly scream with pain and saw her holding the lower right part of her face with her right hand; every few seconds she would yell out because of the pain. She told her coworkers that it felt like a knife was going through the right side of her cheek, and even described feelings resembling an electrical shock shooting through that region of her face. The pains were worsened by any attempt on her part to move her jaw or open her mouth. The only doctor that Lori had been seeing at the time was her gynecologist; therefore Carol, another worker in that office, said, "We need to call Dr. Kassis."

After speaking with Carol, I recognized immediately that Lori had a bad case of trigeminal neuralgia; severe pain was arising in the middle division of the trigeminal nerve, which provides sensation from the angle of the jaw to the skin of the cheek. With the severity of the pain that she was having, I gave orders to Carol to admit her to ICU. I then spoke with the ICU nurse and ordered all of the baseline labs as well as an IV line for fluids and medications, the first one being 10mg of morphine in order to begin to control some of her pain. I told her that I had one patient yet to see in the office, and that I would be there after accomplishing that.

I arrived in the ICU to find Lori lying in the second ICU bed and sobbing hysterically, her right hand pressed against her right cheek. I asked her nurse about the timing of her last dose of morphine. Since it had been an hour ago, I repeated that dose now, and began to get a history from Lori.

Up until that afternoon, she had been well. She had no history of head injury, falls, or seizures. She had noticed no changes in eyesight, smell, coordination, or use of her arms or legs. Bladder function was normal, and she had not had any numbness or tingling in her arms or legs. She reported that she did get an occasional migraine. I discovered no history of familial neurologic diseases; I now began my examination.

Lori's vital signs, including BP, pulse, respirations, temperature and oxygen levels were all normal. Because all of her symptoms involved her facial area, I began my exam at her lower extremities and worked my way up to her problem area. I found no rashes or evidence of arthritis. My examination of her abdomen, heart, lungs, and lymph node revealed normal findings. I next examined her ears and nose, as well as her large temporomandibular joints just anterior to each ear – neither of these was tender with my heavy palpations. The only abnormality that I could demonstrate on her neurologic exam was her severe pain over her right cheek when I lightly touched that area; this worsened on any attempt to open her mouth. Sensation over the remainder of her face, head, and neck I found to be normal. I found no swelling or redness in the region, which might have suggested a dental infection or skin infection.

The trigeminal nerve arises in our brain stem, which comprises the lower part of our brain. In a small cavity on the inside of our skull resides a large collection of nerve cells known as the gasserian ganglion, from which all three divisions of the nerve extend. These three divisions travel in different directions, leave the skull through tiny holes (a foramen), and finally expand in order that they might send the brain sensory messages from the various parts of our face. The ophthalmic division covers the region of our forehead and above the eyes; the maxillary division covers our cheek regions; the mandibular division supplies the region along our jaw line as well as our lower gums. A patient with trigeminal neuralgia will usually experience his or her symptoms in just one of three divisions of the nerve. Compression of a part of the nerve by a brain blood vessel that is not following its correct path is the cause of this syndrome in the majority of its victims; however, in my evaluation of Lori I had to do an MRI of her brain with contrast – both to look for that artery as well as to exclude the presence of a tumor, multiple sclerosis, or a cyst that might compress the nerve. However, no matter how much I might discuss the origin and evaluation of this problem, there lay before me a young woman in agony with her pain, to whom I must now attempt to give relief.

The pain in this disorder arises from abnormal discharges from a particular division of the nerve; it's analogous to having a seizure that involves only one nerve in the body. This discharge may produce a pain so severe that it probably would be difficult to mimic it even by using medieval torture devices. Therefore, over the years physicians have actually used anti-seizure medications in order to control the pains of trigeminal neuralgia – and with reasonable success. Tegretol has been our first-line agent in the fight against this pain, and works by decreasing the nerve discharges that are causing seizures, or, in this case, the discharges in the trigeminal nerve. Often we have to add other antiepileptic drugs to the Tegretol, such as Topamax, Neurontin, Lamictal, and Depakene in order to gain control of the trigeminal discharges – just as we often need more than one medication to combat brain epilepsy. There exists an IV solution of Depakene; however, our pharmacy was out of it on this day. All of the other drugs have to be given orally, and I was staring a Lori, who could not open her mouth easily.

I finally decided on the following plan: I started Lori on high dose cortisone (solu-medrol) in hopes of decreasing the irritation in and around the nerve. Tegretol and Lamictal both come in a tablet that can dissolve in her mouth, while Depakene and Topamax are available in liquid forms. I explained to Lori that, if she could just open her mouth for a couple of seconds, the nurse could slide 200mg of both Tegretol and Lamictal into her mouth, where they would dissolve; if she could tolerate a straw for another few seconds, the nurse would also give her 200mg of liquid Lamictal. Lori made a valiant effort so that we were able to accomplish these tasks. Between these medications and the morphine administered regularly, she was finally able to get a little sleep.

The next morning arrived, and I entered the ICU with a slight feeling of apprehension, wondering if I had made any progress in controlling Lori's pain. I had only received one phone call from the night nurse about her, which I considered to be a good sign.

After making my rounds on the patient in bed one, I entered Lori's room to find that she was obviously a little better. The pains were coming less frequently, and she was able to partially open her mouth before the pain erupted. To say the least, we were both delighted; now I could increase her medications to levels that were truly in the therapeutic range, which should provide even better control of her pains. I continued the Solu-Medrol, increased both the Tegretol and the Lamictal up to a total of 400mg/day, and started oral Depakene at 200mg mg twice daily. It was time to move her out of ICU to a room with a view of the outside world.

Later that day Lori had her MRI of her brain performed, which excluded tumors, cysts, and MS. However, the radiologist felt that there was, indeed, an aberrant artery compressing the trigeminal nerve.

The anticonvulsants continued to do their job so that Lori was ready for discharge after four days. Although I stopped the Solu-Medrol, I continued her on a tapering dose of the oral steroid Prednisone. We agreed on a follow-up appointment in two weeks.

When I saw her back in the office, she was having no pain from the trigeminal neuralgia, but was experiencing severe fatigue from the drug combination. I measured all of the drug levels, which were in their therapeutic ranges. Although I was controlling the trigeminal neuralgia pains, it was obvious to me that Lori would not be able to tolerate the side effects of the medications; with the severity of her attack, I was certainly unwilling to lower any dosages now, for fear that she would relapse. It was time for a neurosurgical consultation in order to see if one of two procedures that these specialists perform for this disease might put Lori into remission. I arranged for a consultation with a well-respected neurosurgeon at the Shannon Clinic in San Angelo.

Neurosurgeons will usually choose one of the two common procedures in their arsenal to treat trigeminal neuralgia. The first of these is known as a "percutaneous rhizotomy," a procedure in which the operator uses radiofrequency applied to the part of the nerve causing the pain in order to destroy that part of the nerve. Since the nerve does not move any of the facial muscles, patients on whom this procedure is performed experience, at most, some mild numbness in the previous area of discomfort. During this procedure, the neurosurgeon passes an electrode through a specialized needle into the gasserian ganglion where he creates a permanent radiofrequency-induced lesion in the chosen portion of that ganglion. The operator may repeat the treatment if the patient's symptoms recur.

Dr. Michael Lorenz was able to evaluate Lori by early September and performed the rhizotomy a week later. She truly got excellent results from the procedure, and I was able to discontinue all of her medications except her Tegretol. I might have stopped that as well, however, because her attack had been so intense, I felt more comfortable leaving her on a low-dose of that drug.

From the time of her rhizotomy in 2003 until October, 2007, Lori's neuralgia remained in remission, and she returned to living a normal life again. But while working one Tuesday afternoon, she suddenly developed the same excruciating pain in the exact location and with the same intensity as in her prior attack. She shrieked both because of the pain and also with the horror of realizing what she was about to have to endure again.

Once again, I admitted her to ICU. After my exam had confirmed the diagnosis once again, I began the same regimen that had worked before to quiet her attack. I called Dr. Lorenz both to notify him that Lori's severe neuralgia had returned and to ask him to reevaluate her as soon as her symptoms had improved; he agreed to do so.

It took five days for the pain to subside enough so that Lori could open her mouth and eat with minimal discomfort. As usual, the medications sedated her fairly significantly; but they certainly controlled the pain reasonably well. I repeated her MRI, which, once again excluded the presence of tumors, cysts, and findings compatible with MS. However, the radiologist still felt that the aberrant vessel was impinging on the trigeminal nerve.

I discharged Lori on Saturday on her medication cocktail, and she saw Dr. Lorenz for reevaluation of her condition on the following Wednesday. After reviewing Lori's MRI scan and listening to her description of these severe episodes of the neuralgia pain, he decided that he needed to operate; the goal of the operation being to move this particular artery away from the trigeminal nerve. He ordered an MR angiogram, which demonstrates the brain vessels better than does a standard MRI, and then scheduled the surgery for the following day. Statistics regarding this microvascular surgery tell us that 70% of operated patients are free of pain and off all medications at ten years – results which are pretty good. A neurosurgeon Dr. James Barker commented in a 2006 *New England Journal* article concerning trigeminal neuralgia that it is his opinion that nearly all patients with this disorder have a blood vessel which compresses the trigeminal nerve; therefore probably all patients with severe symptoms deserve to undergo the surgery.

Dr. Lorenz completed the operation without difficulty the next day, and Lori's recovery was uneventful. Furthermore, she related that her pain in the right cheek was gone. She stayed in the hospital overnight, but awakened the following morning complaining of a pain that began at her right jaw and ran down the right mandibular region toward her chin; it was not as severe as the previous pain. Dr. Lorenz examined her and felt that this discomfort was probably originating from her right temporomandibular joint, which is the large joint located just in front of the ear, and felt that this was due to having the breathing tube in place during surgery. He told her that he expected the pain to resolve. Therefore he discharged Lori on Tegretol and hydrocodone for pain, with instructions to see him next week.

Trigeminal neuralgia is not a rare condition; most patients affected by it have pain that is similar to that experienced by Lori – but which is less severe, relatively infrequent, and responds well to Tegretol or one of the other drugs utilized to manage its pain. Lori's variant of this disorder obviously does not fall into this category; in fact, I would say that – in the era prior to the existence of any treatment options for the disorder of this severity – Lori might well have been one of the suicide victims.

Lori arrived home late that Friday; however, by four AM on Saturday the pain radiating down her right jaw had now morphed into the exact replica of her previous pain, but which now was affecting a different division of the trigeminal nerve – the division that supplies the skin over the mandibular region as well as the lower teeth and gums. My examination, once again, showed that her temporomandibular joint was not tender to my palpation; however, she could barely open her mouth without screaming with pain; there was no evidence of a dental problem; her neurologic examination was normal except for the extreme pain that she experienced when I lightly touched the skin of her right cheek.

I again began the treatments that had been successful before, and repeated her MRI. No new brain lesions had emerged since her last one, the temporomandibular joints appeared to be normal, and there was no sinus infection.

Lori remained miserable over the next two days. Because of this lack of progress, I contacted Dr. Robert Larson, a neurologist in Dallas, who treated a lot of these patients. After hearing the entire story, he responded, "I know many neurologists in this city who could not have treated this woman as well as you have; I commend your expertise." He suggested adding a high dose of intravenous Depakene every 12 hours; however, if I saw no improvement, he would then accept her in transfer to the University of Texas Southwestern Medical Center in Dallas. I called him the next day with her dismal progress report, so I transferred her the next day.

While in the hospital in Dallas, all of the subspecialists who evaluated Lori felt that, having failed in response to the first two surgeries as well as to multiple medications, the next step that they ought to take was "gamma knife" treatment – which involves no knife whatsoever – but, rather, consists in the radiotherapist isolating the part of the trigeminal nerve that he wishes to treat and administering radiation to that area in order to decrease the discharges.

After this was accomplished, Lori was followed by Dr. Larson, who adjusted her medications. Additional flairs in 2012 and 2013 led to two additional radiation treatments in Dallas, which put her disease into remission once again. However, in November, 2013, she developed another horrendous episode of pain in the same region of her face, necessitating my admitting her to our hospital again for treatment. Dr. Larson had written out a protocol that I could follow in order to treat an exacerbation of her disease. After I observed no improvement in Lori's condition over three days, I spoke with Dr. Larson, who said, "There's nothing more I can add."

Within the past year, two new neurosurgeons had been recruited by Hendrick Medical Center in Abilene. I had referred a few cases to one of them, and I was impressed with his expertise. I called their office and spoke with his partner, who agreed to accept Lori in transfer. I told him of all the procedures that the patient had undergone, but that information did not put him off in the least. And so, once again, Lori went to another hospital (which, at least, was closer this time) for evaluation by a man who might be able to approach her from a different perspective.

And indeed he did. After completing his review of all of the data, Dr. Roger Eisenburger called me to tell me that he was going to repeat her rhyzotomy, even indicating that he was a little surprised that the other consultants had not considered that option.

Dr. Eisenburger operated the following morning, and the procedure gave Lori complete relief of her pain within a matter of hours. He and I discussed the medications on which to send her home – finally deciding on Tegretol 400mg twice daily, Neurontin 600mg twice daily, and Lyrica 100mg twice daily.

Lori remained without any major symptoms of her disease over the next two years, and was finally able to function again. I gradually tapered her medications and she now remains symptom free on just two drugs: Tegretol 400mg twice daily and Neurontin 800mg at nighttime. Since I had not been treating her since I retired in March, 2015, I spoke with her just before I started writing this chapter; she is still doing well, with no relapse of her neuralgia.

This fire blazed from the start, almost like the one that ravaged Rome many centuries ago, and it took ten years and multiple consultants in order to put it out; this feat was finally accomplished by getting another "second opinion" from a new consultant. Both Lori and I are thankful that those awful ten years are now history, and that her life going forward looks to be bright and promising.

CHAPTER 12

THE SEEDS ARE SOWN

I have loved practicing medicine for forty years. First of all, I absolutely enjoyed the fact that I was lucky enough to be learning something new almost every day of my existence. However, I felt even more fortunate that I was able to help someone, in some way, almost every day during my working years. I became surprised at how unlucky so many patients are; that the "flying finger of fickle fate" had landed upon them, and that this landing had given them horrible disease processes, which then went on to make their lives miserable. Over the course of many encounters I got to know – not only everything about my patient, both mentally and physically – but also all about their family dynamics; so many times it was just that dysfunctional dynamic that was producing the extreme misery perceived by my patient.

And so, I was my patients' scientific healer, their counselor, almost their priest, and their psychiatrist – all jobs that seemed to be inherent in my being their physician. I loved it when I was able to treat a near-death patient in the ICU, and, through the miraculous workings of medications together with my clinical examination and judgement, bring that patient back to his or her family again. On the other hand, I dreaded having to give a patient the bad news that cancer, or some other incurable disease, had entered their body. Of course I would refer that patient to the proper subspecialist for treatment (most often to no avail). But it was in that moment when I had to essentially take the hope of living away from that person that I felt the most grief. Often the patient, their family, and I would cry together for a while as the news began to settle in on their brains – brains that were full of hope before I walked through the examination room door.

The worst of this kind of episode occurred about 2006. Joe Gotcher had had surgery and radiation for throat cancer about ten years earlier, which seemed to have cured him. However, after those ten years had passed, he came to my office one day complaining of some pain in his left ear region that had been present over the past month – but with no other symptoms. After my exam had revealed no masses in his mouth, throat, ear, or neck, and his chest x-ray was normal, I told Joe and his family that I was still worried about the previous cancer; I referred him back to his ENT specialist for reevaluation.

When I saw him back after the ENT consultation, Joe told me that the doctor had looked down his throat, and had found no evidence of recurrence of his cancer. However, he was still having his pain. At that time I was certain that his cancer had returned, but that we just hadn't found it yet. I ordered a CT scan of his neck with contrast to get a better look at the entire area; and, of course, it was there – a metastasis about a centimeter in diameter located in the left side of his neck.

When he and his daughter returned on the Tuesday following the CT scan, I took his daughter to my office and showed her the report. Crying, I told her that I did NOT want to be the one to give him this news. After considerable discussion, she finally told me that he would, in fact, rather hear it from me than anyone else.

We both entered the exam room. And I sat down on my stool as usual. With the tears welling, I managed to tell Joe what the scan had revealed – that, after ten years of remission, his throat cancer had returned. Joe, a big man of six feet or so, got up from his chair, walked over to me and hugged me, thanking me for being honest with him. We both knew that he was not going to do well – since he had already received the maximum radiation dose at the time of his first diagnosis. Yet, I felt compelled to send him to the oncologist for his opinion. He tried a few courses of chemotherapy, which Joe could not tolerate. Joe died about six months later.

These patients in this small town became like family to me. There were so many that I looked forward to seeing in the office, which was a time for us to catch up on things going on with them, me, and our families. Of course I dealt with their health issues as well; however, there existed a true friendship between us. We often became closer as their diseases took devastating toll on these friends. Often times all I had to offer them was the time that I spent listening to them along with the love and kindness that I tried to give to them. As some of them died (as was inevitable) I would often mourn his or her loss for weeks. I always felt as if I made a difference to people by practicing in a small town; however, I also felt like my patients who died took little pieces of me with them when they passed to the great beyond. Fortunately, they left enough of me around so that I could continue my work.

Jim Bowman was one of those poor souls upon whom that "fickle finger" landed. Jim was a large man, around six feet five inches tall, overweight, who had developed diabetes mellitus about twelve years before I was asked by one of our local doctors to consult on him in the ICU in May 2011. By that time, Jim was on insulin for his diabetes, and had suffered complications of that disease – complications which included a heart attack, diabetic eye disease, and severe peripheral vascular disease (poor circulation going down both legs to his feet). Because of the latter problem Jim had developed a bad right foot infection about three weeks prior to entering the hospital. The bacteria had spread from the foot infection into the bloodstream, which was suggested by the organism's growth in the blood cultures drawn on admission. We call this spread into the bloodstream "bacteremia." Any bacteria may cause bacteremia; however, in this case the laboratory identified the organism as MRSA.

MRSA is a staphylococcus aureus species, which is extremely virulent; once it is in the bloodstream it can land on perfectly normal heart valves, causing an infection that may then spread from the heart valve to other organs of the body. It is also capable of seeding any other part of the body merely by the fact that it is growing in the blood.

At the hospital, the physicians checked for blood clots in Jim's leg (negative), checked the circulation, and felt that circulation was good enough to carry the antibiotics to the foot. Therefore, they decided to treat Jim for two weeks with Vancomycin (an anti-MRSA antibiotic), which should cure both the foot infection and the bacteremia. However, these physicians did not think about the bacteremia or the potential heart valve infection as carefully as they should have. For, with MRSA bacteremia, one has to either prove that the valves are normal by having a cardiologist look at them via a trans-esophageal echocardiogram, or assume that they are infected and treat with four weeks of antibiotic therapy. If the cardiologist sees normal valves, then a two-week course of antibiotics is appropriate.

His physician sent Jim home on a two-week course of Vancomycin intravenously, and then saw him back a few days after that treatment had been completed, at which time the patient's foot infection had resolved, and he was feeling pretty much back to his normal state of health. His doctor arranged to see him back in a month for follow up.

Four weeks went by. Jim then presented to our ER with a two-week history of an aching back pain, which had become unrelenting and was present in all positions. He rated it an 8/10 on the pain scale. So far, he had experienced no numbness or tingling in his legs and no difficulty with urination. He stated that he had felt a little feverish on a couple of occasions, but did not take his temperature. He was still able to walk up to the time of admission, and had had no neck pain, chest pain, or abdominal pain; he said that his blood sugars had been doing well.

The ER physician had done routine lab work on the patient, along with x-rays of his chest and lower back. The latter showed some arthritis, but nothing else remarkable. He had called our family physician who was on "ER Call" for that day, who decided, because of Jim's severe back pain and his other medical problems, to admit the patient to ICU. After completing his examination of Jim about an hour after his arrival in the ICU, he asked me to see him because he was unsure of the diagnosis. When I got this call, I immediately called the ICU nurse and asked her to try to get the records from the other hospital in town where he had been admitted before for my review; I finally arrived in ICU to evaluate Jim around 7:30 that night.

After arriving in the ICU, I sat down to review the previous hospital record along with the current lab values and x-rays. Jim's white blood count was minimally elevated at 13,000 (normal up to 10,000); his kidney function was still normal. X-rays of his lower back showed the arthritis of a seventy-four year old man, but nothing more. The records from the other hospital definitely documented the presence of an MRSA bacteremia at that time; however, those records did not show any evidence that a cardiologist had seen the patient or that a four-week course of antibiotics had been considered by his admitting physician. I gathered my neurologic tools, and entered room 1 – introducing myself on the way in. As usual, I pulled a chair toward his bed, and sat down to listen to his story.

I saw that Jim was a large man, filling the ICU bed completely. He was lying on his left side. "This is my most comfortable position," he said, "but, even with me lying this way, the pain is still awful." He related that his pain had begun fairly quickly; over a matter of two to three days it had reached its maximum. Moving in any way would make the pain worse – even when he was lying down. Jim described the pain as a very bad "ache"; when I asked him to point to the involved region, he pointed to the lower thoracic portion of his spine located just above the lumbar spine already imaged. The patient told me that he had not experienced any radiation of the pain into the lower abdomen, groin, or legs, nor had he felt any numbness in those regions. He now had a catheter in his bladder; however, he told me that he had still been able to urinate normally up to the time of this admission.   Jim related that if he sneezed or coughed he would experience a "God awful" spasm in the muscles of his back that were near the source of the pain.

I next proceeded with my exam of the patient. His vital signs were normal, as were the examinations of his head (without fundus exam), neck, lungs, and abdomen. I saw no skin rash that would suggest the presence of "shingles." His circulation to his legs certainly was abysmal; however, I saw that his infection had healed.

My neurologic exam demonstrated no focal weakness in arms or legs; as expected because of his diabetes, his sensation in his feet was markedly diminished. He exhibited no abnormal reflexes; the sensation in the anal area was normal.

I saved the most important parts of the exam for last: I listened to his heart in all positions, and heard no abnormal sounds or murmurs. Then I had Jim sit up on the edge of the bed, and I proceeded to palpate and to percuss rather forcefully each vertebra of his back, beginning from the neck and working my way all the way down to his tailbone. When I reached the region of the lower thoracic area, Jim gave out a loud shout of pain when I percussed vertebral numbers T9 and T 10. "That's it," he said. "That's the spot; man that hurt."

I now knew that this was not an ordinary back pain like we all get. It was present constantly – even in the supine posture -- aggravated by coughing and sneezing, and the involved area was exquisitely tender to percussion. With the prior bacteremia, I strongly suspected that this man had infection in his vertebrae that were seeded from that bacteremia.

I ordered three sets of blood cultures along with a sedimentation rate and CRP – the latter two being measures of inflammation. I started Jim on Vancomycin to be started as soon as the blood cultures were drawn, and scheduled him for an MRI of his thoracic and lumbar spines with contrast to be done ASAP in the morning. I slightly increased his dosage of morphine to give him better pain control through the night.

The following morning Jim underwent an MRI study of his entire thoracic and lumbar spine, with the addition of contrast; the latter helps the radiologist see areas of infection and malignancy more clearly. Within an hour after the scan had been completed I received a call from the radiologist, who was in the process of interpreting the study. Dr. Donald Richter told me that there, indeed, was infection present in vertebrae T 9 and T10, but that the disk separating those two vertebrae was also infected. However, the truly bad news was that the infection had spread to the epidural space surrounding the spinal cord in those areas, forming an abscess which was just beginning to put pressure on the spinal cord traversing that region. If this process were allowed to progress, the enlarging abscess would, ultimately, compress the spinal cord so much that Jim would be a paraplegic – unable to move his legs or control his bladder function. That morning's sedimentation rate of 132mm/hour was also consistent with this kind of infection.

With this new information, I called his admitting physician to let him know the dangerous condition affecting Jim's back and also to tell him that I was going to transfer Jim to the neurosurgeon in Abilene, who would drain that abscess in order to relieve the pressure on the spinal cord -- thereby aborting the potential paraplegia.

Because this problem constitutes a neurosurgical emergency, I had no problem arranging Jim's transfer to our favorite neurosurgeon; within an hour the patient was on his way to Hendrick Medical Center for further management of his problem. Prior to the transfer, I sat down and explained to Jim and his family the nature of the problem and why surgical drainage of the abscess would be necessary. I showed the MRI scan to the family, so that they could have a better understanding of the problem; Jim and all of his family understood the reason for the neurosurgical consultation.

I would like to say that my diagnosis of this rare condition (affecting about two in 10,000 persons) led to a favorable outcome, and that Jim went on to do well. Unfortunately, that happy ending did not occur in this case.

After arriving at Hendrick Medical Center, the neurosurgeon evaluated Jim, reviewed the scan, and agreed with the diagnosis. Since Jim had not experienced any radiation of the pain around to his lower abdomen or into his legs, the consultant felt that, with Jim already covered with Vancomycin, he would plan surgery for the following morning. This surgery would include drainage of the epidural abscess, debridement of infected bone, and the obtaining of cultures from all of the infected areas. However, around 1 AM the following morning Jim complained of numbness in his legs; within thirty minutes he was unable to move his legs at all. In spite of the neurosurgeon operating on Jim within the hour, he remained a quadriplegic from that time forward. The blood cultures that we drew from Jim on his admission to our hospital once again grew MRSA, indicating the presence of that bacteremia at the time of his admission. The cultures obtained by the neurosurgeon at time of operation all grew the same organism.

This case demonstrates definitively just how virulent MRSA is, and why we treat even the smallest of skin wounds infected with this bacteria so aggressively. Jim's initial infection with MRSA was in his right foot; but the organism spread from there into his bloodstream, most likely even prior to his first admission to the hospital. Since our blood flows throughout our bodies, the MRSA bugs were able to seed Jim's vertebral bone with infection, an infection that then spread across a disk and into the adjacent vertebra. Ultimately, the infection then spread from those regions into the epidural space, thereby causing the epidural abscess to form. I would say that the MRSA bacteremia occurred very early during the course of his foot infection, during which the vertebra became infected. After completing the inadequate two weeks of antibiotic therapy, the infected vertebra then seeded his bloodstream again – giving rise to the positive blood cultures that we saw at our hospital. I propose this mechanism because a cardiologist actually performed a trans-esophageal echo while Jim was at Hendrick, during which he observed normal heart valves. This time Jim was treated with six full weeks of IV Vancomycin antibiotic therapy in order to be certain that the vertebral bone infection (osteomyelitis) would be cured.

I would see Jim in our hospital off and on over the years when I would be covering for our group over a weekend. His diabetes, with its complications, remained fairly stable over the years, but the paraplegia persisted – a reminder to me to always be meticulous in my review of laboratory data and its interpretation and to always treat MRSA infections with the great respect and caution that they deserve.

CHAPTER 13

THE ART OF RURAL MEDICINE

I always knew that I did not wish to practice medicine in the city. My time spent in the seminary in Northern California, where I was surrounded by luscious green farmlands, a small, working ranch next door, and the Eel River – our swimming and fishing site – less than a mile away, created a memory in me that haunted me as I went through all of my training. During that training I always studied the material in such a manner that might prepare me for rural practice, where I would not have subspecialists around upon whom I could "dump" complicated cases. I never ended up in an area quite as beautiful as was the Northern California site; however, both Rupert, Idaho, and Sweetwater, Texas, had their own special beauty. Each was in high desert areas and were surrounded by large swaths of farmlands; the farmers in Idaho grew potatoes and sugar beets, while the Texans grew cotton and raised cattle. In Idaho, my family and I could drive for two hours, camp by the Salmon River, and fish for trout for dinner. Sweetwater was surrounded by cotton fields for miles, so that one had to drive much further for any water sports. However, Sweetwater possessed a great clinic, with six physicians, and a wonderful fifty-four bed hospital, where the staff gave great patient care. Each location greatly contributed to the clinical expertise that I developed over the years, expertise which showed itself at its best during my practice in Sweetwater. However, it was during my practice in Rupert that I gleaned invaluable knowledge –

some of which came merely because I found myself in medical circumstances in which I HAD to do something, or the patient would die, while I acquired the rest of it via my extensive reading of the medical literature and from interaction with my surgical colleagues.

For example, during my first year in Rupert I was called one afternoon to the ER to see a nine-month-old boy, whom the nurse had told me was not breathing well. I arrived to find that this child was blue from lack of oxygen and totally limp; a child who had, basically, given up on trying to breath. "Oh shit!" I muttered to myself as I gazed down at this dying infant. I was sweating and my heart pounding at this point. I had no experience whatsoever in handling this kind of situation in a child. An arterial blood gas that had been drawn just prior to my arrival showed that his pCO_2 was 137 (normal being around 28.), while his oxygen level was only 40 (normal being 96). I very gently opened his mouth, and was able to see his swollen epiglottis blocking his airway.

Dr. William Hansen happened to be in the ER at that time. "Have you ever done a tracheostomy before?" I asked. When he replied "No," I told him that I had never done one either; however, I must do one now, or this child would die. I asked him to help me, and he readily agreed.

After cleansing the skin of his neck, I localized the trachea (the main windpipe), and, using a small needle, I gently placed that needle into the trachea. Using that as my guide, I made a small incision in the skin; with tiny forceps, and then gently separated the muscle tissue below the skin until I could see the trachea. Passing a suture around the trachea, I now, at least, had control of his windpipe. I next made a small x-shaped incision in the trachea to create an opening for the small endotracheal tube that I had ready. The moment of truth had now arrived; if I didn't get the tube into the trachea, this child would die in my arms. All of the ER nurses along with Dr. Hanson hovered around the gurney, each one holding their breath. Very gently, I placed the end the tube on top of the incision in the trachea and started to apply pressure; there was a little resistance at first, but after a few seconds, the tube slipped into his windpipe. Directing the tip of the tube slightly downward into the trachea, I quickly inflated the balloon which keeps the tube in place; we attached a breathing bag to our end of the endotracheal tube, and started air compressions. I listened to both lungs, and heard air flowing on both sides; we had done it. All of our anal sphincters relaxed a bit at this point! As we bagged the patient, the boy started looking pink again, which fact told us that air was truly reaching his lungs. I ordered a portable chest x-ray to check the tube placement; the tip of the tube was in perfect position.

I called Dr. John Gunderson, the ENT specialist in Twin Falls, to inform him that a nurse and I were bringing this child to the ER there and asked him to meet us. The forty-minute trip to the hospital seemed like an eternity to the nurse and I; however, we were encouraged by the fact that the boy demonstrated a little movement as well as by the fact that he was no longer limp and blue. As we arrived in the ER, Dr. Gunderson was there, and took over the management of this very ill child. He commended us on our work, noting that without our intervention, the boy would surely have expired. The boy recovered from his severe epiglottitis over the next week; in fact, his mother brought him to my office about two weeks later, by which time he was thriving. I was ecstatic!

However, as I will discuss later, much of my new knowledge came from my surgical colleagues, knowledge acquired as we managed the trauma cases together, and when they would ask me to scrub in on an elective case being performed on one of my patients.

When, fresh from residency training, I started my solo practice, I had no idea that, over the next three to four years, I would be exposed to clinical situations in Rupert that I never would have dreamed about during my formal training. In fact, I would say that, during my thirteen years of practicing in Rupert, I expanded my medical knowledge by at least threefold over that which I had acquired during my residency training. And so on to another example …

In studying to take my board exam, there was one page in *Harrison's Textbook of Medicine* (my main study source for that most memorable exam) that mentioned "other viral diseases," among which was described "Orf ." This is a skin disorder acquired from sheep, in which that patient develops a large (1 & 1/2 inches), purple skin lesion, usually somewhere on their hand or arm. As I read over this page dozens of times in preparing for the boards, I remember telling myself that I would never see this disease.

Rupert proved that I was wrong about that within the first two weeks of my practice there, when Dr. Don Pates (a family physician) called to tell me that he had a gentleman in his office who had a very large, raised purple lesion on his right wrist. I told Don to send the man right over to my office, so that I could look at the lesion ... and you are correct – the patient had "Orf." When I called Don to explain this to him, his only reply was, "Orf, Orf to you, too!" I actually ended up seeing about six more cases during my thirteen years in that town. Fortunately, the skin lesion goes away by itself in about two weeks, and there is no scarring process involved in the process.

At the time that I arrived in Rupert, the hospital was bereft of both a CT scanner and an ICU. Our "ICU" consisted of a room with a monitor. About three years later I was able to form a committee, which ran a community campaign to raise money to build an ICU. Some of that money raised was matched by federal funds, so that we were able to design and build a very adequate four-bed Intensive Care Unit.

There were two surgeons serving the hospitals in Rupert as well as the Cassia Memorial Hospital across the Snake River in the town of Burley. Each had served in Viet NAM, and both were experts in their specialty. Both of them had dealt with every type of trauma imaginable while they served in a medivac units over in 'NAM. I developed a close working relationship with each of them, by referring patients to them, by doing consultations on their patients, and, lastly, by scrubbing in on their surgeries if they needed help.

In addition to finding out that I had to see children as part of my duties at the hospital, I quickly discovered that, due to our proximity to I-84, our hospital received a fairly large number of trauma patients in our ER. Now, general internists are not trained in the management of the trauma patient during their residency. So, when at first, these mangled bodies would appear in our ER, I would simply order oxygen, all of the baseline labs, EKG, get a chest and abdomen x-ray along with x-rays of whatever bone didn't look right, start two large IV's, and call for the surgeon. Most had multiple injuries, and ultimately the surgeon would take them to the OR for further management. Prior to that, however, the surgeon might have to spend time putting a chest tube into each lung space to drain any blood that might have shown on the chest film, thereby improving the patient's breathing. Performing those procedures took time, thus delaying the definitive treatment of the patient's injuries.

I decided that I needed to quickly learn how to manage trauma victims more efficiently, and in a way that would be of some help to the surgeons. I ordered a critical care textbook, and began reading the chapters as fast as I could. As I read it, I learned quickly that there are conditions that can affect trauma victims that are totally unfamiliar to the general internist and the family doctor; conditions involving the various internal injuries and how to diagnose them and conditions involving the upper airway and lungs, which could easily kill the patient before he or she might even have a chance of making it into the OR. I read extensively about head injuries – their mechanism of brain damage, the physical exam findings associated with them, and the various methods for lowering elevated pressure inside the skull. I learned that there are differing amounts of blood loss around a bone fracture, with blood loss from a femoral bone or pelvic bone fracture being of a considerable volume when compared the loss related to other fractures. Lastly, I read about the different procedures that needed to be done to stabilize the heart and lung status of the patient, so that the patient might go to surgery. These procedures included the different methods of intubation of the patient, the placement of a chest tube into the pleural space (the space between the lung and the chest wall) to remove air and/or blood, the different ways in which to place a large IV into the main veins of the patient, and how to do a diagnostic "peritoneal tap" of the patient's abdomen to see if there was an internal injury (remember, we did NOT have a CT scanner).

After I finished reading the tome and reviewing it, I sat down with Hayden Ellingham, a surgeon, and discussed how I might be of more help to him in these cases. We talked about what I had learned; I told him that I now felt comfortable enough to be able handle the heart and lung and airway problems, thereby allowing him to concentrate on the internal abdominal injuries along with the orthopedic trauma. I had, however, never put a chest tube in before; I asked if he would teach me that procedure, a request to which he readily agreed.

The opportunity to learn how to perform that operation came soon enough; one of my emphysema patients developed a hole in his lung when a "bleb" opened up, letting air from the lung flow into the pleural space. This condition is known as a "spontaneous pneumothorax." With this problem, the patient experiences sudden chest pain along with a marked decrease in his ability to breathe; if the pressure inside the chest cavity rises excessively, then blood flow through the heart stops, and the patient dies.

I called Hayden, who had just finished doing a case in our OR; he arrived in the ER in just a few minutes. After we had gathered all of the necessary equipment, Hayden talked me through the procedure. After I had anesthetized the skin and ribs on the left lateral part of the patient's chest, I then made an incision in the skin large enough to allow a small chest tube to enter; using some fairly large forceps (these are like long needle-nosed pliers) I spread the muscles of the chest until I entered the pleural space – at which time I heard air exiting. I covered the hole, grabbed the end of the already lubricated tube with the forceps, and guided the tube with the forceps through the chest muscles until it entered the pleural space -- directing the tube up toward the top of the patient's lung. After removing the forceps, I continued to advance the tube upward until only about six inches remained outside of his body, at which time the nurses then connected the tube to the suction apparatus. After putting petroleum jelly around the tube at its entrance into the chest, I anchored the tube in place with tape, placing tape all around the entrance site – tape which overlapped the chest tube. Inspection of the chest tube drainage receptacle revealed proper functioning of the tube. More importantly, the patient was breathing much more easily and now had a normal oxygen level. Lastly, Hayden and I reviewed a portable chest x-ray, which showed us that the chest tube was in its proper position. My lesson was now complete.

I admitted my patient to the hospital to wait for the leak in his lung to heal. Normally this process takes about three to four days, and is recognized when I no longer see bubbles in the receptacle's water seal when the patient breathes. At that point, I clamp the tube and recheck his chest x-ray the following day. If the lung has remained expanded, then I can safely discontinue the chest tube, rechecking the chest x-ray one last time on the following day in order to be sure that the lung has truly healed. In this situation, I had placed a small diameter chest tube. In a trauma patient, in whom one expects to find both air and blood in that space, I would place a tube with a much larger diameter so that it would be able to drain the blood.

And so, over the years, I would manage the problems in the upper part of the trauma victim, while either Dr. Hayden Ellingham or Dr. Leo Brown cared for all of the other injuries that might be present. With multiple cases upon which to practice our coordination of care, we arrived at a point where we could have that patient stable enough to go into surgery within a relatively short time. And remember, we were it for that patient. There was no air ambulance services back then; our closest larger hospital was sixty-five miles away by ground travel. Cardiac and neurosurgery consultants were respectively 250 and 80 miles away. Thus, we were the doctors who might possibly have a chance to save these trauma victims.

Before returning to my Sweetwater narrative, I have to discuss the survivor of the worst trauma case that we cared for while I was in Rupert.

It was late February, 1978. A thirty-six year-old gypsum plant worker had finished his shift around five PM and was heading home on his Harley. It had snowed slightly three days before, and the temperature had not risen enough to remove all of the patches of ice from the roads. Richard Thompson had ridden his Harleys for many years and felt comfortable riding in this kind of weather. As he was crossing the intersection of West Baseline Road and 100 West, a pickup going South hit one of the ice patches, so that the driver could not brake effectively enough to avoid sideswiping Richard on his motorcycle. The pickup had been traveling at a speed of fifty mph; so that Richard and his motorcycle were a mangled mess.

A homeowner living at that corner saw the accident and called 911. Since Rupert is a small town, the ambulance arrived quickly, scooped up Richard, and got him to our ER within fifteen minutes.

The nurse recognized immediately how critical the situation was, and promptly called me and both Drs. Ellingham and Brown to come immediately. I arrived first, and found one of the nurses vainly trying to place an IV into a vein in Richard's right arm – a vein that, with the patient's non-existent blood pressure, was no longer usable. I gazed down at the patient lying on the gurney; his color now resembled that of the sheet beneath him. His breathing was shallow and he moaned off and on. I placed an oral airway (a device to keep the tongue from obstructing the windpipe), and started him on 100% oxygen with a mask. Then I asked the nurses to get me the kit that would have everything necessary for me to place a large IV catheter into the subclavian vein – the large vein that runs just beneath the collar bone and which returns blood to the heart. Among other things, this man needed the placement of the catheter so that we could give him both IV saline and blood; hoping that the administration of the fluids would raise his blood pressure to a level compatible with life. I briefly examined Richard, while the nurses prepared the equipment.

Richard had obviously suffered a severe head injury and was comatose; however, his eyes moved about randomly, which indicated the thinking portion of his brain may yet be functional. His heart rate was 124/minute and percussion of both sides of his chest revealed dullness – indicating that there was probable blood in the chest cavity.

By this time, Dr. Ellingham arrived to evaluate the patient. At that moment I was in the middle of placing an IV catheter into Richard's right subclavian vein in order to be able to give him the fluids and blood as rapidly as possible. Dr. Ellingham ordered the nurses to get two chest tube kits ready, along with the setup for a peritoneal lavage. (In the latter procedure the surgeon places a dialysis catheter into the patient's abdomen. If frank blood is present on entering the abdomen, then the surgeon knows immediately that there are damaged organs inside the abdomen. If there is no frank blood appearing, then a liter of saline is quickly infused into the abdomen; the saline bottle is then placed on the floor, so that the infused fluid will return, which is then sent to the lab to have the number of red blood cells in it counted. If the number of cells is above a certain value, then the surgeon has to assume that there are internal injuries; so that he must explore the abdomen. (Nowadays we just do a CT scan to look for internal injuries but at that time none was available to us.)

By now Richard's portable chest x-ray and lateral neck x-ray had both returned, showing blood in both pleural spaces and a small pneumothorax on the right, along with two fractured ribs on each side. There was no obvious neck fracture. Therefore, before intubating his windpipe to control his airway, I quickly placed a large chest tube into the right side of his chest, which immediately drained about 1.5 liters of blood. Richard's oxygen level increased from 83% up to 89% with placement of the tube; however, that level would not be adequate. Furthermore, I was dealing with an unconscious man who could not protect his airway. Therefore, after giving him an IV dose of Ativan, I slipped an endotracheal tube (breathing tube) into his trachea, and placed him on the ventilator in order prevent aspiration of material into his lung as well as to provide Richard with adequate oxygen delivery. A chest x-ray confirmed that the end of the tube was in proper position.

Dr. Ellingham had already placed the abdominal catheter, and the fluid was in the process of returning to the bottle. He had ordered x-rays of the patient's abdomen, pelvis, and both legs. While we waited for these results to return, I placed the second chest tube into the left chest; like the one on the right, it too shortly drained a liter of blood from the left side of Richard's chest. A portable chest x-ray again confirmed good chest tube position.

Dr. Brown had arrived by this time, and, as the results returned, we all reviewed them. Here was a patient hit by a pickup, who was still in shock after three bottles of saline and two units of packed cells (blood); who also had (at the very least) a brain contusion producing coma, bilaterally broken ribs with blood and air in the chest cavities, internal injuries as confirmed by the cell count on the returned fluid, and fractures of his tibia and fibula in both of his lower legs. His EKG showed no heart damage. Currently, his heart rate was 110/minute, and his blood gases (measuring oxygen and carbon dioxide levels) were good.

The OR crew had already been called in by Dr. Ellingham; now it was time to take him to surgery. Dr. Brown planned to put in another subclavian IV line after they got him into the OR in order to be able to give Richard more fluids and blood to improve his blood pressure further and get him out of shock. However, only their repair of the internal organ damage would ultimately save this man.

What these two experienced surgeons found as they entered Richard's abdomen was impressive indeed. He had a ruptured liver and spleen, which had bled about three liters of blood into his abdomen, along with a tear in his left kidney. They removed the spleen and repaired the liver and the torn left kidney.

After closing the abdomen, they then turned their attention to the fractures in both legs. Both bones in the lower legs were broken and displaced; so that the surgeons had to realign them all and fasten them in position with plates of metal secured with screws placed into the bones.

After almost four hours, they finally finished the operation, and Richard was taken first to the recovery room, and then to room 102 – just across from the nurses' station. His blood pressure was now stable at 116/70, his heart rate normal at 104, and he was tolerating the ventilator via a rare dose Ativan to sedate him while the machine breathed for him. I repeated all of his labs and also an electrocardiogram as soon as he arrived in the room. His blood count now showed an hemoglobin of 10, normal electrolytes – but his kidney function had suffered because of the shock and the muscle injuries. However, the most worrisome of the results was his electrocardiogram, which now showed evidence of injury. This most likely represented cardiac contusion due to the chest trauma that Richard suffered in the wreck (it would be as if someone had hit the heart with a baseball bat, causing a bruise). The CK value (muscle enzyme level) had actually fallen from a value of 850 in the ER to 300 at the present time. (At that time, we did not have the laboratory technology to separate heart muscle damage from ordinary muscle damage).

I got a cot and placed it in Richard's room so I could monitor him. A cardiac monitor traced his heart rhythm, and I had the nurses place the heart defibrillator on the left side of his bed ... just in case. The EKG changes definitely made me feel uneasy.

Things went well until around 2:30 AM, when the monitor alarm sounded; when I looked at his rhythm, I saw that his heart had gone into a very lethal rhythm known as ventricular fibrillation. I called the nurses, who charged the defibrillator, and then I delivered the charge to Richard's heart. There was a pause on the monitor, then his heart resumed its normal rhythm once again. Because of this episode, I gave Richard a rapid dose of Lidocaine and then started him on a drip of Lidocaine – a drug used to prevent such episodes. However, these episodes of ventricular fibrillation occurred off and on throughout the night, so that I ended up having to shock his heart back into rhythm thirteen times. The last episode happened around 8AM, after which time his heart rhythm remained stable.

Over the next week Richard remained stable. I placed a feeding tube to nourish him, placed him on an air bed, and gave him medicines to prevent blood clots. However, though his neurologic exam did not suggest a localized area of brain damage, he remained comatose. I spoke with my neurosurgeon, Dr. Peter Schloss in Pocatello, early on during that week, but Peter did not think that Richard was yet stable enough for transfer. Finally, at the end of the week, I spoke to Peter once again, and indicated that Richard's vitals, lab work, heart and lungs had been stable for the last three days – yet I still had a comatose patient who desperately needed a CT scan of his brain in order to visualize its damage and to assess the patient's prognosis. Peter agreed to accept him in transfer the next day.

The following morning we copied all of Peter's hospital records and gathered all of his x-rays; a nurse and I rode the seventy-five miles with Richard to the Pocatello Medical Center. By the time of transfer, he no longer was ventilator-dependent, but could breathe on his own through the endotracheal tube with just oxygen added.

I met Dr. Schloss for the first time that day; we had spoken on the phone for a number of years, but had not had a face-to-face encounter. After admitting Richard, he performed a CT scan of his brain, which – surprisingly – showed only diffuse brain swelling (a contusion – something from which he should gradually recover). Dr. Schloss asked the orthopedic and surgery specialists to follow Richard's other problems, while he and his neurology nurses managed the contusion.

From what I heard, Richard was in the hospital for about two weeks, and then went to a rehab facility for further physical therapy. I heard nothing more about the case after he went to rehab.

However, this tale did not entirely end for me until 1984, when a man in his forties now entered my office in Rupert and asked the receptionist if he could speak with me. The receptionist, responding as usual, told him that I was running behind, and that he may not be able to see me. He responded, "I AM not leaving here without talking with Dr. Kassis; I also think that he might like to see me." So my receptionist called me out of a room to tell me of the dilemma. I asked her to send the man back to my office and that I would see him there.

He arrived in my office a few seconds later and introduced himself. "Dr. Kassis, my name is Richard Thompson. You may not remember me; and, having lost memory of a number of months of my life back in 1974, I certainly have no recollection of you. However, I have been told by a number of people that you were primarily responsible for saving my life back then. I came here to thank you for that. I spent a lot of time in Pocatello doing physical and mental therapy.

After my release, I moved to Tempe, Arizona, where I have some family, attended college, and then went on to veterinary school. I have been practicing veterinary medicine now for the past two years. I thank you for making all of this possible for me."

I was shocked and overwhelmed. Being a "crier," a fact which everyone who is close to me will verify, I felt tears well up as I managed to get out, "I certainly do remember you, and you are truly very welcome. I AM so glad – first of all that you survived the ordeal – and that you have been motivated to pursue your profession. I AM so happy that you returned to see me. It's nice to know that I win one periodically. I offer you best wishes in your future life and career."

And with that visit, I truly realized that my presence in a small rural town actually made the difference between life and death for many of the inhabitants; as I went to work every day, this fact continued to give me the greatest feeling of accomplishment in the performance of my chosen profession.

So, as we leave the discussion of my early learning process, one can begin to realize that the somewhat unique expansion of my education did not merely come just from reading the *New England Journal of Medicine* weekly (although I did read the most pertinent articles – usually on Sundays). Rather it came from a number of sources – sources which the average internist is not ever exposed to. Nowadays most students are trained on dummies, while they obtain an inadequate knowledge base by answering multiple choice questions in their textbooks instead of by reading articles about the diseases and their management -- facts about disease processes that they truly must memorize and actually know. On the other hand, I had a twelve-week hematology clerkship at UC Davis Sacramento Medical Center, which was followed by a twelve-week rotation with my own beloved family physician. Not only was he was a very accomplished family doctor, he was one of the kindest men whom I have had the pleasure of knowing. He reinforced for me the importance of taking a thorough history from the patient. He also spent time teaching me how to inject almost every joint and bursa in our bodies – a skill which most of today's practicing internists and family practice doctors lack entirely.

The critical care textbooks that I have read over the years have made me competent in my care of the critically ill patient; and, lastly, my exposure in Rupert to the surgeons' knowledge and their literature definitely expanded both my procedural abilities as well as my differential diagnosis of a patient's potential problems. My expertise in this area of intensive care medicine was definitely the most valuable thing that I had to offer the rural towns. I also found that, over the years, as the cases appeared, I had to improve my knowledge of neurology. All of this medical knowledge, which was acquired in rather unique ways, definitely allowed me to be most effective during the last fifteen years of my practice in Sweetwater. And so I return there now for the discussion of the next case in which the embers were once again glowing.

CHAPTER 14

THE BALLERINA'S

WAYWARD LEG

I walked into one of my examination rooms in April, 2009, to find a lithe and lovely, twenty-six-year-old women. About five feet six, and weighing only 115 pounds, she sported short brown hair and brown eyes. She had on a blue blouse, with pressed grey pants – obviously a woman who knew how to dress. At first glance, she appeared to be the embodiment of good health. And, indeed, on further questioning, she impressed me even further with her efforts to remain healthy; she ate nutritious food, and exercised extensively – in fact, she was a ballerina, who was in constant demand for performances as far away as Dallas.

I sat down on my stool and began to obtain her history. As I listened to her tale, I quickly became aware that there was certainly nothing wrong with her heart, nor with her lungs. She spent hours in training without experiencing any shortness of breath, chest pain, or fainting episodes. Shirley, as she was known, did not even complain of any arthritis symptoms, which one might expect with her long hours of practice. No, she had developed a different sort of problem altogether.

She told me that, while she was rehearsing in Dallas about two- and-a- half months ago, she had fallen during one of the dance moves in which she had to jump and land on her left foot. It almost seemed to her as if the leg just gave way as she landed. Fortunately, she suffered no injuries, and was able to go on and finish the ballet with the rest of the ensemble.

She was scheduled to perform in Swan Lake at the Bass Auditorium in Fort Worth and had begun rehearsals three weeks ago; however, as she rehearsed, she was beginning to feel as if she couldn't control her left leg as well as she could during performances in Dallas. She was most aware of the problem when she did her spins; she felt that these were just not as "tight" as they had been a few months before. Shirley had not noticed a problem performing her day-to-day activities, which even involved her ascending the stairs to her second-floor apartment The patient had developed no headache, blurred vision, dizziness, difficulty speaking, swallowing or hearing (symptoms which would suggest a problem in her brain). Neither had she noticed any difficulty with her arm and hand strength, nor with her overall coordination. Lastly, Shirley had not experienced any numbness or tingling sensations in either her arms or her legs; she had no family history of any neurological disease. The patient had noticed no unusual smells at the performance hall and had never experienced a seizure. She managed her finances without difficulty. The only medication that she regularly took was a multivitamin.

Shirley had studied ballet for many years –which had finally begun to pay off about three years ago when she began to obtain regular roles in various ballets in Texas. The child of a single mother, Shirley had scrimped and saved her money in order to pay for her ballet lessons. She finally landed a scholarship with the Texas Ballet Theater in Dallas, where she proved to her instructors that she definitely had talent. During the last week prior to this visit she had tripped while walking down the sidewalk – her left foot merely seemed to "catch" on the walkway. It was this last episode that had prompted her consultation with me today. She was in Sweetwater visiting her mother, one of my patients; it was the mother who had recommended that Shirley see me concerning her symptoms.

Finally pleased that I had obtained a satisfactory history, I got up from my stool, handed her a gown, and stepped out of room while she disrobed to the waist; I also asked that she remove her stockings in order to facilitate my neurologic exam. My nurse and I reentered the exam room a few minutes later; and, with Shirley sitting on the exam table, I began the exam.

Her vital signs were all normal. I made sure to check her blood pressure first with her lying down and then after she had stood by the exam table for two minutes. I do this in order to assess whether her bodily fluid levels are normal as well as to see if her neurologic system responds normally to such a dramatic change in position (there should be less than a 10 mm of mercury drop in pressure between the two positions).

My examination of her head, neck, lungs, heart, abdomen, skin, and joints revealed normal findings. The neurologic exam took much longer. The function of both the thinking part of her brain as well as the lower, automatic portion was normal. She could clap her hands at a good pace, which suggested normal coordination.

I next tested the strength of her arm and leg muscles, which I found to be normal. However, when I asked her to tap her feet against my hands, her left foot performed slightly more slowly than did the right, while her hands performed this maneuver normally. I could easily have written this off to the fact that she was right-handed; however, my subsequent exam findings made this slight slowing more significant.

Because I had to perform a very detailed examination of her different modes of sensation, the entire neurologic examination took me forty minutes to perform. After all of this time, I discovered only one other subtle but significant finding, which simply was that her left great toe lifted ever so slightly upward when I stroked the bottom of her foot with my pen. This reflex is normally present when we are infants, at the time when our brain has yet to establish its connection to the spinal cord. If found in an adult, this sign (Babinski's sign) indicates that the brain is again losing its connection to the spinal cord as that cord travels from the base of the skull down to the lower back -- a journey which permits our brain to control the legs. Unless I find other localizing findings (such as arm or leg weakness), the fact that this abnormal reflex is present merely tells me that a problem exists somewhere along the course of the cord. Something was interrupting part of her brain's messages to the neurons that controlled the movements of her left foot and leg – an interruption that not only was disturbing her dancing prowess, but which seemed to be now affecting her walking ability. From my examination, I had no idea if this lesion was a tumor, multiple sclerosis, a herniated disc (these are quite rare in the thoracic region of the back – occurring in only one out a million people), or some form of infection. Nothing in her story or in my examination suggested that the brain itself was involved in this process.

After Shirley had finished dressing, I sat down with her and, with the aid of models, explained to her my suspicions, indicating at the same time that we would need to do an MRI of her entire spine to firmly establish the diagnosis and to get her to a neurosurgeon who could manage the problem. I explained to her that the "neurological rule" in cases such as hers was that, because my examination could not precisely localize the site of the problem, we were obligated to image the entire spinal cord. She understood fully; so that I arranged for my office to schedule the MRI of the spine with contrast for the following Thursday, with follow up in two weeks. I told her to curtail her dancing until we had a diagnosis.

I saw Shirley back to review her MRI results two weeks later. In the meantime she had begun to experience a somewhat dull, aching pain that radiated from her back in the mid-chest area partly around her left side toward the upper abdomen. She rated the pain level at 3/10; it had not interfered with her activities, nor had she developed any fever or chills. The pain was worsened by changing positions – especially during the night. She had noticed no other new symptoms.

I sat down on the chair next to her and pulled up her MRI report on my laptop. There was no mention of tumor, MS, or infection in the report. Instead, the radiologist described the presence of a herniated disc that was located at the intervertebral disc between her T6-T7 vertebrae. This herniation was partially compressing the left side of her spinal cord at that level, thus producing her difficulty controlling her left leg and foot. This was great news; for, with surgery, she had an easily correctable problem.

Everyone talks about the discs that are present in our backs; but just what are they? I believe that most of us have, at some point in our lives, opened up a golf ball to see how it is made. What we found was a bunch of rubber bands wrapped tightly around an orange rubber ball; all of this was then placed inside of a hard shell. The discs, which act as cushions between our vertebrae, are similarly made. They are truly disc-shaped, with the outer part (the annulus) consisting in multiple layers of strong fibers, which surround an inner gelatinous core ("the nucleus pulposus"); it's this latter part that provides the cushioning effect for us.

A patient develops a "herniated disc" when the outer fibers of the disc break down and allow the gelatinous core to "herniate" through them. Since the space in the spinal canal is fixed, that core ends up "bumping" either into the spinal cord or into one of the nerves that are leaving the cord to go where they are needed. The herniation in Shirley's case produced just enough pressure on the spinal cord that her brain was having difficulty getting its message to her left leg and foot – thus producing the subtle motor problems that she was experiencing together with the very subtle neurological findings that I found on examining her. The fact that she was now experiencing pain at the site of the disc herniation meant that the herniation had worsened, and was now pressing on the nerve root exiting that part of her spinal cord. Because most of our back's motion involves the neck or lower back, these are the regions where most herniated discs occur. Because the herniated core tends to impinge upon the nerve roots exiting the back in those regions (and does not involve the spinal cord as much), this type of patient complains of severe pain radiating down the arm or the leg (sciatica). Even though physicians are asked to use fewer narcotics, this is one type of discomfort which definitely demands a short-term course of narcotics in order to give the patient some relief.

Having diagnosed her problem, I now had to have the neurosurgeon remove the offending disc. Nowadays the surgeons are able to do this via a small incision as an outpatient procedure, with minimal down time. Since her mother lived in Sweetwater, Shirley elected to have her surgery performed by my favorite neurosurgeon in Abilene. After I called him, he agreed to see her on the following Tuesday and operated that the following Thursday. Because of the strenuous activity involved in her profession, he did not allow her to return to work for a month. However, upon her return, Shirley continued to blossom as a ballerina. Her mother kept me apprised of her progress.

So, again, we see a disorder begin as an ember – this time a very small one, with very subtle symptoms at first, but which worsened during the week prior to the patient's revisiting me to review her MRI results. If she had experienced a significant fall during the weeks before her visit, Shirley could easily have ended up a quadriplegic. The two subtle neurologic findings might easily have been missed had I performed a more cursory exam; however those exam findings led to the performance of the proper imaging procedure, which then lead to a correct diagnosis and proper treatment. I AM once again reminded of the old rule in medicine with which I would, invariably, harass my students: "When all else fails, examine the patient."

CHAPTER 15

EMPATHY AND EMBERS

Over the years, I have heard patients talking with their friends about their physicians. Of all of the complaints that I have overheard, two stand out as being the most common and meaningful for the patients. The first, and most common complaint voiced by these people was "My doctor just won't take the time to listen to me," while the second most common one was "My doctor doesn't seem to empathize at all with me concerning my problems." A third, but much less common gripe voiced by these people was "My doctor acts like he's God, and nothing that I say means anything to him." I feel that these are all valid complaints against those persons who have chosen Medicine, a profession in which a person dedicates oneself to the art of healing an ill person, but who have chosen to practice that art in a somewhat half-hearted or self-serving manner.

As I have mentioned previously, my extensive reading of the Sherlock Holmes mysteries taught me how important a patient's history is in directing me toward the correct diagnosis; ninety-five percent of the clues to that diagnosis lie hidden in that person's narration of his or her symptoms; so it behooved me to learn to listen very attentively, asking pertinent questions if I felt that I needed more clarification. I applied the art of "active listening" to the process of my obtaining a history from my patients, an art in which I would repeat to them what I thought I had heard them tell me; so that the person would have the chance to be certain that I had understood them correctly. The ability to listen to patients, I had gleaned through the perusal of literature; my ability to empathize with my patients came about through my having been a patient many, many times in my life beginning when I was an infant.

Having been born with a cleft lip and palate, I had undergone three surgeries to begin the repair of this defect by the age of five. Since I was an infant during that time, I have no recollection of those early procedures. However, at age five my parents took me back to Minneapolis for a forth surgery, of which I still have a vivid and horrible memory.

I remember meeting with the surgeon, who, apparently, was the doctor who had performed the prior procedures. I can recall his explanation to me of the planned surgery, "I AM going to fix a hole in your mouth"; that was it – no explanation of what I was about to face, the pain that I might experience after the procedure, or any details about how the operation was to be performed. (I guess that he thought that a child of my age was incapable of understanding such things.). At that point, my parents took me to a surgical floor, placed me into a crib, and left. I remember feeling fearful, uninformed and abandoned. Although only five years old, I was a bright kid; certainly, I could have understood what was to happen to me had the surgeon or his nurse bothered to explain some of the details to me.

I will remember the next morning forever. I was wheeled into the OR, lifted onto the operating table, and the nurse placed an IV into my left arm. At that point my "hell" began. Two nurses held me down, while a third nurse placed a mask over my mouth and nose. Soon I began to smell and taste the Ether anesthetic, which the anesthesiologist had begun to drip onto the mask to induce anesthesia. The ether is an irritating liquid, with a pungent and nauseating smell, from which I could not escape. Because the drug acts slowly over seven to ten minutes before it induces anesthesia, I became frantic, fighting the nurses with all of my strength -- but to no avail. Relief finally came as I drifted into unconsciousness. This entire scenario haunts me to his day.

The surgery having been completed, I spent my time in the recovery room vomiting for God knows how long (that's the Ether again.), before finally being moved back to the surgical ward. My mother was there; my Dad just couldn't deal with all of the bandages and blood on my face. I immediately noticed that the nurses had placed arm restraints on me, so that I could not touch my face. I remember saying to myself "If you believe that I AM going to touch my face after what I have just been through, then you are all idiots." I would require further revision surgeries during my late teenage years, all of which were easy to cope with compared to this early torture. The doctor performing these later operations was an exact clone of Bob Newhart of TV fame; he proved himself to be not only a very capable reconstructive surgeon, but also a gentle human being.

Indeed, I was to have encounters with many surgeons and medical doctors throughout the rest of my life; so that I became familiar with how patients react as they go through testing procedures, multiple doctor consultations, and the intense pain which can result from various surgical procedures. I experienced the anxiety that one has while waiting for the doctors to make up their minds about a diagnosis -- the fear that this time that diagnosis may be some form of cancer instead of a benign process. I truly developed empathy for the patients whom I would be treating for the rest of my career.

But now I must move on to the embers that I mentioned at the beginning of this chapter. Indeed, I had a disorder which acted like the some of the disorders that we have already explored throughout this narrative – a disorder whose embers would barely flicker for years, but then erupt into a blaze which would periodically make my life miserable; however, the flames would then regress to their flicker once again, and my symptoms would disappear. (It reminds me of Erica's situation.) For twenty-one years this obscure disease affected my life.

I actually started out to be a priest, spending my high school years boarding in a minor seminary. It was during this time that my disorder attacked me on two different occasions. Each time the symptoms were the same; I experienced a severe pain in the upper part of my abdomen, which was a burning, hunger-like sensation, and which might last for one to three days. The worst episode attacked me after I had gone to bed one night; it was so severe that I walked the floor all night praying that it would resolve. I never developed fever, chills, nausea, vomiting, nor any radiation of the pain to my chest or back. The pain finally eased by around five AM, and I was able to go to sleep; however, I was left with some residual pain for about three days. I did not complain to anyone about this problem for fear of being labelled a "wuss."

By 1957 I had decided that the priesthood, with its vow of celibacy, was just not for me, so that I decided to pursue a career in Medicine. I had been impressed by some of the physicians who, through their dedication and expertise, had helped me to approach life with a measure of self-confidence. Having always entertained a desire to help people; I thought that, as a physician, I would be able fulfill that goal. I applied to the University of Santa Clara for my pre-medical studies, and was accepted. During my four years at the university the embers of my disorder remained in a smoldering state, and I had no acute attacks over that period.

In September, 1966, I matriculated to Loyola-Stritch School of Medicine in Chicago, which at that time was located across the street from Cook County Hospital, the institution in which we did all of our clinical work during our third and fourth years of training. Although the training was arduous, I found that I loved medicine, and was willing to put in the long hours which were required of me in order to learn the material.

It was midway through my first year as a medical student when I experienced the worst attack of the abdominal pain that I had ever had. The pain was so bad that I could not stand upright, because to do so made the pain almost unbearable. I was afraid to see a physician for fear of falling behind in my classes.   Had I been in my third year of medical school, instead of my first, I would have recognized that this symptom indicated that the lining of my abdomen was being severely irritated by an inflammatory process (such as acute appendicitis), and that a surgeon really needed to operate on me in order to explore the abdomen, find the cause, and fix it. I had what is known as a "surgical abdomen"; I was extremely lucky that I did not become deathly ill from this process. I continued taking Maalox and refrained from eating very much during that week, and finally the pain resolved. I continued with my studies.

After graduating from Loyola-Stritch, and completing my residency in Internal Medicine at UC Davis School of medicine, I began my practice in Rupert, Idaho in 1975. A few months passed, and I became very busy, with little time off. I did manage to see Dr. John Stewart a Gastroenterologist in Twin Falls about my problem, who felt that my symptoms were the result of gastritis (an inflammation of the stomach lining); he placed me on a regimen of Prilosec to suppress the amount of acid that my stomach, with a follow up in six months. He seemed to have no interest in evaluating me for gallbladder disease, which could cause periodic flares such as I was having, nor did he feel the need to perform an endoscopy on my stomach

As it happened, one of my colleagues agreed to cover the 1976 Christmas Holiday for me, giving me a grand total of three days off, which I would be able to spend at home with my family. We were all ecstatic, especially my boys. We finished wrapping all of the packages, watched movies, and generally enjoyed the time together.

On Christmas Eve, we went to bed around eleven, knowing full well that we would all be up early on Christmas morning. However, I was awakened around five AM with a horrible pain located in the middle of my abdomen, similar to my previous attacks – only this time it was worse. It was a very sharp pain without any radiation and unassociated with fever, chills, cough, nausea, vomiting, or diarrhea. My trying to breathe or to move around greatly worsened the discomfort. Once again, I could not stand up straight without having the pain intensity worsen.

My wife lay next to me; I did not want to awaken her this early, nor did I want to destroy the boys' Christmas celebration. Lying there, I palpated my abdomen; merely percussing the area where I felt the pain caused me to wince with the increased level of pain produced by that minor maneuver. Yes ... I definitely had a "surgical abdomen"; I knew then that Dr. Ellingham, who was on call this Christmas, would find himself inside my abdomen later that morning. In a way, I was relieved that the flames had, again, begun to worsen in intensity and that now Dr. Ellingham would be able to diagnose this smoldering mystery which had given me such grief off and on for over twenty years.

The boys arose at six-thirty; Joan and I made coffee and then we settled into our usual living room chairs to watch the boys open their presents. Clothes, of course, were never a hit; but this year we had gotten most of the toys correct. Marc and Jeremy were pleased with their Christmas "loot." Looking at all of the torn and scattered wrapping paper, a person would surmise that we had given the boys everything that was available at Walmart.

It was now time for me to tell Joan that I would most likely be going to surgery later today; that I was calling Dr. Ellingham to ask if he would meet me at the ER to evaluate my abdomen. She was NOT happy. "Why couldn't you have told me this sooner?" she chided. I explained my reasoning for not doing so; which explanation she blew off entirely. I told her that I would see Dr. Ellingham, and then call her to let her know what was going on. She seemed a bit happier with this plan; so I got into my car and travelled the five-minute drive to the hospital.

Hayden was waiting for me when I arrived. He had already ordered the CBC, CMP, amylase, cardiac enzymes, chest and abdomen x-rays, and an EKG. While Nancy the head ER nurse started an IV, Hayden took my somewhat convoluted history, and then examined me. The only part of the exam that he found to be persistently abnormal was the abdominal exam, during which he definitely demonstrated findings consistent with irritation of the abdominal wall – indicating that he needed to explore my abdomen. He mentioned that, with my previous episodes resembling this one, he was surprised that I had not gotten into serious trouble before this.

The x-rays did not suggest a perforation of a hollow organ, and my white count was elevated to 15,700, which merely suggested inflammation. The EKG and amylase tests were normal. Dr. Ellingham had already called in the OR crew, so it was not long before Marilyn was wheeling my gurney into the OR. I had called Joan to let her know what was happening; she told me that she would see me when I came out of recovery.

I have never figured out why hospitals are kept so cold – especially the operating Rooms. I was shivering so badly that I was unable to crawl onto the operating table without help. With the three nurses and the Nurse Anesthetist helping, I finally managed to get into a comfortable position. Sarah, the Nurse Anesthetist then put a mask over my face through which she now ran 100% oxygen for a few minutes, which elevates the oxygen level in my blood, thereby giving her significant leeway should she have any difficulty placing a breathing tube into my windpipe. Now came the familiar burning of the bolus of IV anesthetic medicine as it made its way up my veins. My next recollection is my awakening in the recovery room; the nurse continuously saying "We're all done, Dr. Kassis; everything went fine."

As I regained consciousness, I became aware of a painful and very obnoxious NG tube traveling through my left nostril, down into my stomach. This tube is used to suck drainage from my stomach and intestine to keep them from accumulating fluids which would then put pressure on the area where the bowel is sewn together. By now I was also aware of a very bad, sharp pain that ran down the middle of my abdomen from the umbilicus to my pubic bone; this would be the surgical incision, which currently hurt like hell. My first words were "I need something for pain." I was able to doze off and on after Marilyn gave me the wonderful Morphine; and, after spending about an hour in recovery, the nurses moved me to a room on the Med-Surg floor, where I would remain until discharge. Sally the "charge nurse" told me that Dr. Ellingham had found a "Meckel's Diverticulum," and had removed it, along with my appendix. She said that he would be in to see me in the morning, and would explain more then.

For all those years, I had been suffering symptoms that were caused by complications of a Meckel's Diverticulum, which is nothing more than the persistence of a proximal part of the vitelline duct -- a duct which brings nourishment to the fetus while in utero. By the time of the birth of the infant, this duct should have atrophied and disappeared – never to rear its ugly head again. Yet this is the most common congenital malformation of the gastrointestinal tract, persisting in about 2% of the population, and producing symptoms in one of two ways:

First of all, since it protrudes from the colon like an "extra appendix," the diverticulum can get "sucked" into the colon, which then pulls it along toward the rectum. We call this "intussusception." The portion of the colon which is trapped inside of the healthy part rapidly loses its blood supply; so that the patient with this condition may then experience severe abdominal pain along with bleeding from the GI tract. If not diagnosed, the loss of the circulation to the trapped bowel will, ultimately lead to sepsis and death.

In other cases, the lining of the diverticulum becomes populated with gastric (stomach lining) cells, which manufacture gastric acid. If the tip of the diverticulum ruptures, the acid then released irritates the adjacent tissues and produces significant inflammation. Fortunately for me, our abdomen contains a large apron of fatty tissue known as the "omentum," which is mobile and is attracted to areas of inflammation that occurs inside of the abdomen – thus "walling off" the inflammation or infection. Indeed, this fatty apron had already saved me from disaster many times leading up to the current episode. Because many of the diverticula do contain acid-secreting cells, a Meckel's Diverticulum may be looked for by performing a radiological "Meckel's Scan," which can visualize the acid-producing cells. However, that test is only positive in 60% of cases -- in the ones that truly have the most number of the gastric cells present. Looking at the scan will be seen the Meckel's Diverticulum lighting up on the film.

In my case this was not a time to consider performing a "Meckel's scan"; I had acute abdominal pain, rebound tenderness, and an elevated white blood count. Neither Hayden nor I doubted that surgical exploration of my abdomen was necessary – both to obtain a diagnosis and to fix the problem.

The next morning Dr. Ellingham explained to me that he had opened my abdomen, and ultimately found the Meckel's diverticulum located at its usual position – two feet from where the large and small and large intestine meet. The two-inch long diverticulum had ruptured at its tip, allowing leakage of gastric acid into the surrounding tissues. He also found evidence of prior rupture, with lots of scar tissue surrounding the diverticulum, scarring which extended into the adjacent "omentum." He had carefully removed about eighteen inches of the small intestine containing the diverticulum, and sewed the two ends of the intestine back together. Because he did not want any increased pressure at the sites of the bowel anastomoses, he told me that I would have to tolerate the nasogastric tube for five days. (Having that tube in place was miserable, while the incisional pain was minimal by the third post-operative day.) Finally, on the fifth day, the nurse Allison entered my room carrying gloves and a basin; I knew then that she was about to remove this alien thing from my body, and I rejoiced accordingly.

Two more days in the hospital as Dr. Ellingham advanced my diet; then I was home free. The fire was out once and for all, and there were no more embers that might spark another episode.

And so these embers with periodic fires had persisted (as did Erica's embers and flares had done) for over twenty years. A gastrointestinal specialist whom I saw failed to even consider a Meckel's Diverticulum as a diagnosis (nor did he seem to be interested in pursuing even other, more common diagnoses.) During the remainder of my career as an Internist I made this diagnosis in six more patients -- a diagnosis which I was able to make predominantly by carefully listening to the patients' histories; demonstrating, once again, that Sherlock was right about the necessity of just sitting and listening to the patient, especially one whose disease embers lay dormant much of the time. As my history might suggest, I have never had difficulty emphasizing with my patients and their problems.

CHAPTER 16

ART VERSUS SCIENCE

With the arrival of the Affordable Care Act and the electronic medical record also came "algorithms," which were designed by people of the insurance companies (including Medicare) who are of the firm belief that every patient must fit into one of these algorithms for diagnosis and treatment purposes. Medicare even has gone so far as to penalize hospitals if certain complications happen to a patient during his or her hospital stay.

For example, nowadays every patient admitted to a hospital receives some form of care designed to prevent the development of blood clots in the legs, which might then travel to the lungs. The medical literature supports the facts that, while such preventive treatments are effective, their use WILL NOT assure that clots will be prevented in 100% of the patients receiving them. The severity of the disease affecting the patient, co-morbid conditions (such as the presence of heart failure, kidney disease, levels of coagulation factors, the mobility of the patient) may, in combination, lead to the failure of the preventative procedure or medication – with the result that a blood clot might occur in that patient; this necessitates additional medical treatment and time in the hospital. In that case, Medicare will simply deny payment to the hospital for that additional care; Medicare tells the hospital that the clot simply should not have occurred – even though the medical literature does NOT support such a thought process. These are the kind of people that your physician has to deal with on a daily basis, both in the office and the hospital.

And so we now have the pigeonholes into which members of the insurance industry believe that patients must fit into if they are to be able to receive both the testing necessary to make a diagnosis and the treatment needed to manage their problem or problems. Sometimes an insurance representative will simply tell your physician that he doesn't feel that the test is needed; and deny its performance. If you appeal, then your doctor might have to speak with another "insurance physician" (who may not have practiced for a few years, who is not in your doctor's specialty, and has not spoken with or examined your patient), who may still deny the performance of the necessary test – or tell your physician that he can do a less informative exam.   In addition to the time spent with you in the examination room, your physician and his staff now spend a considerable Amount of their time each day dealing with these frustrating conditions in their attempt to deliver your medical care --- and it is only getting worse.

Most disease processes have a pattern as they progress within a patient; hence the importance of the history in trying to diagnose these illnesses. After the physician has obtained the history from the patient, he or she will then often order certain tests designed to confirm the presence of a suspected disease. Sometimes the first test does not confirm that the disease is present; so that the physician may need to order another test, which looks for the disorder in a different manner. If the diagnosis has still not been confirmed, that patient's physician may then seek a second opinion from a specialist; however, even after that consultation – and perhaps even after further testing -- the doctors' suspicion of the presence of a particular diagnosis may still be high, but they have not proven its existence. The science of medicine just hasn't helped them.

In the 1980's Dr. Joseph Sapira first wrote another one of my favorite Physical Diagnosis books, *The Art and Science of Bedside Diagnosis*. As its title indicates, medicine is not a strict science such as is physics. There is a subtlety that exists in the practice of medicine; that subtlety resides in the history of the patient's disease process which he or she supplies to their physician. The next two people whom I AM about to introduce to you demonstrate, once again, a disease which, not only smoldered before its flames became more obvious, but which defied the science of medical practice as well.

Jim Freeze had lived in Rupert, Idaho, for about eighteen years, working for the local sugar beet processing plant for most of that time. He was a large man of about 280 pounds, muscular, and had lost most of his hair by the time I first met him in 1978. Jim had developed both hypertension and elevated cholesterol levels around 1970, which had been poorly controlled over the years – mostly due to the fact that he failed to take his medication much of the time.

I initially encountered Jim in our ER in Minidoka Memorial Hospital as he lay on the gurney looking pale and frightened. At this time the hospital had not yet built its more spacious ER, so there were three nurses, myself, and Jim crammed into a relatively small room. One nurse was in the process of starting an IV in Jim's right arm, another was doing an EKG, while the third nurse wiped the sweat that was pouring from his head and torso. He moaned about the horrible pain he was experiencing in his chest, which had begun about a half-hour before he decided to come to the ER, and which had been associated with one episode of vomiting before calling the ambulance. The nurse handed me the EKG, which demonstrated obvious heart injury across the front wall of his heart, so Jim was having a fairly large heart attack. His history did not suggest any warning chest pains (angina) over the last few days, nor did it suggest that his problem was related to a primary lung or abdominal problem. His blood pressure was elevated at 198/100 in both arms, pulse 110, and respirations 22. When I listened to his lungs, I heard the early buildup of some fluid backing up because of the damaged heart. (This was confirmed by the portable chest x-ray performed in the ER). The pulses in his extremities were equal, and I found no swelling in his legs that would indicate some long-standing heart failure.

I quickly gave him morphine for pain, aspirin, and Furosemide (a medication to remove excess fluid from the body via its action on the kidneys). Because of the rapidity of the action of that drug, Julie, one of the nurses, inserted a catheter into Jim's bladder. After transferring him to the ICU, I added other medications both to protect his heart and to lower his blood pressure. At this time the closest interventional cardiologist was 230 miles away in Boise, and there was no air ambulance system in place. Therefore, my goal was to stabilize Jim's blood pressure, relieve his pain, and treat the buildup of fluid in his lungs as the myocardial infarction evolved. (Treatment today, of course, is much different from what it was in the 1970s.)

By the following day, Jim's pain had resolved, and his condition had stabilized; his blood pressure was normal, and his lungs were now clear. Both the EKG and the levels of his blood cardiac enzyme levels confirmed that he had suffered an occlusion of one of the main vessels supplying the entire front wall of his heart, the resulting loss of oxygen delivery having destroyed much of that heart muscle. The effect is similar to having a pump that can move a liquid at five quarts/minute, whose efficiency suddenly drops to an output of three quarts/minute. When a drop in heart output such as this occurs in a patient's body, tissues lose their normal supply of oxygen delivery and begin to malfunction, manifested by accumulation of fluid in the lungs, difficulty thinking clearly, and the loss of valuable kidney function.

So by that morning I knew that one of Jim's major coronary arteries was clotted off. Questions remained -- could it be re-opened or bypassed ... and what was the condition of the other two arteries that bring blood to the heart? I called my favorite cardiologist Don Stott in Boise, who agreed to take him in transfer. Fortunately, Jim had not had a problem with extra heartbeats with his heart damage, so I felt safe in transferring him to Don that day via ambulance with an ICU nurse riding with him.

Jim arrived safely at Saint Luke's Hospital after a three-and-a-half hour ambulance ride. He had not experienced any more chest pain, and his heart rhythm had remained stable. Don evaluated him as soon as Jim arrived in the ER, admitted him to ICU, continuing the medications that we had begun in Rupert. The next morning he took Jim to the cardiac catheterization suite, where he performed a complete cardiac evaluation, which included injecting dye into all three of the coronary arteries as well as into the cardiac chambers; thus he was able to assess the remaining function of Jim's heart muscle as well as the status of the other two vessels supplying blood to his heart.

The news was not good. As expected, the vessel supplying the front wall of the heart was totally blocked; however, each of the other two arteries demonstrated 90% blockages as well. The myocardial infarction (heart attack) had reduced the pumping ability of Jim's heart from greater than 50% (normal) down to 35%. If either of the remaining two arteries were to become occluded, Jim would either die or progress to intractable heart failure, which would lead, ultimately, to a slow death. With this information now known, Dr. Stott consulted Bob Marsh, a cardiothoracic surgeon, who reviewed the catheterization films, and decided that he would need to perform coronary bypass surgery on Jim if there were to be any hope of preserving the remaining cardiac muscle strength. Bob was the most experienced cardiac surgeon in Boise – performing four to eight of these procedures weekly. Throughout my years in Rupert both he and Don took meticulous care of my cardiac patients. I could not have asked for better. Whenever I would call Don to transfer a patient, his response would always be "Send them up." He never asked, as some other consultants would, whether the patient had insurance; he would just say, "I'll see the patient as soon as they get here."

The surgery went well, but the subsequent years were not kind to Jim and his heart. The damage from both the coronary artery disease and his longstanding hypertension led gradually to the development of intractable congestive heart failure, with his ejection fraction (the measure of the heart's pumping ability) falling to 12%. His cardiac physicians referred him for a heart transplant, which he was able to receive in 1984.

Jim tolerated the transplanted heart well, and had no major problems with the anti-rejection drugs. His diabetes was a little harder to control because of those medications; however, with adjustments in his insulin dosages, I was able to manage that task.

In May, 1986, Jim came to me complaining of abdominal pain, which he had been experiencing for about a month. The pain was classic for gallbladder disease – located just below the right ribcage, dull, and made worse after he ate anything. The pain would increase in intensity beginning about twenty minutes after the meal, radiate around to the right side of his back, and – sometimes – he would have some brief nausea associated with it. This description will be found in any textbook or journal article in which the author is discussing gallbladder disorders. These symptoms usually result from the formation of stones inside the gallbladder, which then irritate the lining of that organ. When the gallbladder contracts after we eat a meal, a stone may then lodge at the exit of the gallbladder; the continued contractions of the gallbladder in the face of the blocked duct produce the pain that the patient experiences after eating – the pain resolving only when the stone dislodges itself from the gallbladder exit (known as the cystic duct).

After I had taken Jim's history, I was convinced that his abdominal problem was the only issue that we had to further evaluate. He had seen his transplant physician two months earlier, who had made no changes to Jim's medical regimen. I began my examination, which confirmed that his cardiac status was perfectly stable; his blood pressure was perfectly controlled, and I found no evidence of cardiac failure.

I began my examination of Jim's abdomen in the lower left side, far away from the area of his symptomatic area; gradually, I worked my right hand around his abdomen until I reached his right upper quadrant. He experienced no discomfort as I lightly palpated the region; however, when I began to push more deeply into that area of the abdomen, Jim said, "Stop. That really hurts." I finished the examination of the rest of his abdomen, and then checked his rectum so that I could check his stool for the presence of blood; none was present. Thus, after completing my evaluation of Jim's presenting complaint, I was now totally certain that all of his symptoms stemmed from a diseased gallbladder and that he would need, in the near future, to part company with that particular organ.

The gallbladder is part of our "biliary system," and is merely an egg-shaped container with muscular walls that stores the bile that is continuously secreted by the liver. When a person eats something, the walls of that container contract to empty the bile from the gallbladder, sending it first through the cystic duct (tube), then through the common bile duct (to which the main duct of the pancreas also connects), and finally through a small opening in the wall of the intestine located just beyond the stomach – the part of the intestine known as the duodenum. Here, both the bile acids and the pancreatic enzymes mix with the recently ingested food so that it might be absorbed further down in the intestine.

Gallbladder "disease" is usually due to the precipitation of stones in the liquid bile being held in the gallbladder, stones that can then irritate the lining of the gallbladder, get stuck at the exit of the gallbladder (at the cystic duct), or – if small enough – travel all the way down through both the cystic duct and the common bile duct and, finally, lodge right at the opening into the intestine. Anytime the flow of bile is halted by the mechanisms just mentioned, bacteria can then enter the stagnant bile and cause it to become infected. Thus, a blockage at the level of the cystic duct can give rise to an infected gallbladder, while a blockage at the entrance to the intestine may allow both the gallbladder and the liver to become infected. The true danger of either type of infection is that the bacteria may then enter the bloodstream, by which they then spread throughout the patient's body, leading to organ failure and death. A small stone might pass all the way through all of the ducts and enter the intestine; however, in so doing it may transiently raise the pressure in the pancreatic duct high enough to induce inflammation in the pancreas (acute pancreatitis), which by itself can be a deadly disorder.

So far Jim had complained only of symptoms of what is known as "gallbladder colic" -- pain brought on when the stone lodges temporarily in the cystic duct and then dislodges itself after the gallbladder stops contracting. Therefore, infection had not yet become an issue. With Jim maintained on a number of medications to depress his immune system in order to prevent his rejection of the transplanted heart, any local infection could easily overwhelm his defenses and quickly lead to a bloodstream spread of the bacteria to the rest of his organs, ultimately leading to his death. Therefore, my job now was to quickly confirm the diagnosis and then get Jim to his transplant team, so that they might then consult the general surgeon to remove the diseased gallbladder.

The day that I first saw Jim for this problem was a Monday. I drew the blood needed for analysis that afternoon; by late Tuesday morning I had the results of his abdominal sonogram, the test which looks for the presence of stones in the gallbladder. It was normal. The radiologist called me to let me know that the pancreas, liver and gallbladder (including the thickness of the gallbladder wall) all appeared to be totally normal.

I immediately scheduled Jim for a nuclear medicine scan of his liver and gallbladder for the following morning. In this test a radioactive tracer is injected into a vein, and the tracer is then taken up by the liver, sent to the gallbladder, from which it then drains into the intestine. If the gallbladder lights up during the test (as it should if there is no stone at its opening), then the technician gives the patient a medication that causes the gallbladder to empty. A normal test will demonstrate the tracer in the liver, the gallbladder, in the ducts, and ultimately in the intestine. After having been given the medicine to induce emptying of the tracer from the gallbladder, the result should be in the 35% to 75% range. Jim had this test performed at 8 AM that Wednesday; I received a call from Bill Larson the radiologist at 11:30, who told me that the scan was normal. At lunchtime I went to the hospital and reviewed both studies, finding – as the radiologist had described – that, indeed both evaluations were normal.

I called Jim and told him that, in spite of the normal study results, I was absolutely convinced that his gallbladder needed to be removed, and that I would be speaking with his transplant physician in Boise later that afternoon. I told him to pack his bags in expectation of traveling to Boise within the next day or so.

As the day neared an end, I put in a call to Bill Fisher, Jim's cardiac transplant physician. I told Bill of my conviction that Jim was having attacks of gallbladder colic, but that our studies thus far were cold stone normal. I expressed my concern that the attacks over the last month were frequent enough that I felt the best thing to do was to quickly get Jim back up to him, so that he could have his gastrointestinal and surgical specialists evaluate the situation. Bill agreed, and arranged for Jim to be admitted to the hospital the following afternoon. I then called Jim and gave him the news.

It was a week-and-a-half later when I received a call from Dr. Fisher regarding Jim Freeze. He told me that every specialist who evaluated Jim at Saint Luke's agreed with me that he needed his gallbladder removed. They repeated the studies that I had done; the gastroenterologist consultant even used a scope to sample the bile that was draining into Jim's intestine so that it could be analyzed – all of these studies were normal.

Finally, they decided that – in spite of normal studies – this man needed to go to surgery. Bill related to me that the operating surgeon told him that he removed a gallbladder from Jim which was one of the most diseased specimens that he had ever seen. The gallbladder walls were thickened by chronic inflammation to the point where they were almost immobile; the inflammation of the gallbladder walls had caused adhesions (scar tissue) to develop around the organ, which made it difficult for him to remove it. He found a number of small stones upon opening up the gallbladder itself.

Considering that the surgeon had to do a standard gallbladder incision for this operation, Jim recovered nicely from his surgery and was discharged by day eight post operation. When I saw him back in the office two weeks later, his cardiac status was perfectly stable, and he still had some minor incisional pain; however, the pain which had been related to his diseased gallbladder was now absent. Jim was still doing well in 1987, when I left Rupert to join another practice.

And so we see here a patient who did not fit into an algorithm, whose symptoms smoldered and flared, and periodically put him at great risk because of his disease, especially when combined with his immune deficiency. The science in this case proved to be unreliable; so that, as Dr. Joseph Sapira sets forth in his book, all of us physicians involved in this particular case had to rely on the "art" of medicine in order to treat Mr. Freeze appropriately. The next case that I will discuss will similarly demonstrate this concept, but in a patient living in Sweetwater, Texas, 1,007 miles away from Rupert, Idaho.

I spent the last fifteen years of my medical career practicing with six other physicians in a small clinic in Sweetwater, Texas. During this time I had the opportunity to follow Kathy Bower over a number of years. Because she was basically a healthy woman in her fifties, I didn't see her very often. One Thursday afternoon in 2011, Kathy appeared in my exam room after having been absent from the office for quite a while. She told me, "I just have not felt well during the last four months. I AM nauseated most of the time. I don't have much of an appetite; and, when I do eat something, the nausea seems to get worse for a while. I've taken Zantac and Pepto-Bismol, but that hasn't seemed to help. I haven't had any pain anywhere in my belly, and I have not thrown up or had any diarrhea."

As I questioned Kathy further, I ascertained that she had not had any fever, chills, cardiac symptoms, or symptoms suggesting any urinary problems. She was on maintenance treatment for hypothyroidism and took some occasional Tylenol for knee arthritis. She had not vomited any blood nor noticed any in her stools. She had no history of hypertension or diabetes, and had had a normal colonoscopy about a year ago and a complete hysterectomy many years prior to this visit. I began my examination.

Kathy stood at 5 feet, 3 inches, and weighed 188 pounds. She had brown hair, which fell to her shoulders, and was dressed in blue jeans together with a plaid blouse. She appeared obviously worried about her symptoms. Her blood pressure, pulse, breathing, temperature and oxygen levels were all normal. As I examined her from the head down through her lungs, I neither saw, felt, nor heard any abnormalities. My nurse lifted up her gown so that I could examine her abdomen. As with Mr. Freeze, I began my exam on her lower left side, and gradually worked my way around her abdomen – first gently percussing it, and then palpating more deeply. All was well until I pushed into her abdomen just below her right ribcage; as I pushed my examining fingers downward, she grimaced and said, "That hurts." With my hand still in the same position, I asked her to take a deep breath. As she breathed in, she suddenly stopped and yelled "Ouch. That really hurt." I removed my right hand from her abdomen, and let her relax for a minute. I then completed the rest of my exam and stepped out of the room so that Kathy could get dressed.

Upon my return to the exam room, Kathy was still complaining a bit about the pain that I had caused her. I brought up the pictures of the abdomen on my computer and began to explain to her my conclusions regarding her symptoms and my exam; I thought all of her symptoms were due to chronic cholecystitis, which is an irritation of the lining of the gallbladder. I told her that the pain that she experienced when I examined her was classic for gallbladder disease; for, as the irritated gallbladder descended while she took a deep breath, it finally touched my examining hand, contact which caused her immediately to have more pain. I explained that I needed to evaluate her for other problems that might cause her symptoms; therefore some blood tests, x-ray tests, and even an endoscopy of her stomach lining would all be needed in order to complete that evaluation, lest I miss another disease process that was actually making her miserable. After she had listened to my explanation and reviewed the pictures, she agreed to proceed with the workup.

That day I drew labs to look for anemia and to check her liver and kidney function along with levels of her pancreatic enzymes and a test for celiac disease. I also drew blood to check for the presence of bacteria in her stomach known as H. pylori, which can cause inflammation in the stomach, ulcers, and can even lead to the development of stomach cancer. I had my nurse schedule her for an abdominal sonogram and for a consultation with the surgeon Dr.

Waltham. She would be the person who would do the endoscopy of the stomach and any surgery that might later be needed. Kathy would follow up in two weeks, by which time all of these things would have been accomplished. I started her on Omeprazole just to decrease her stomach's acid secretion while the workup proceeded.

Two weeks went quickly by, and Kathy returned once again to go over all of the results of her testing. Unfortunately, she was still having the same symptoms as before, with no relief from the Omeprazole. I quickly re-examined her abdomen, and elicited the same findings as on my previous exam. Then we sat down and reviewed all of her test findings.

All of her blood work was normal. The abdominal sonogram showed a normal liver, gallbladder, and pancreas. On endoscopy the esophagus, stomach, and duodenum were seen by Dr. Waltham to be normal. Both the blood test drawn in the office and the stomach lining biopsies obtained by Dr. Waltham revealed the absence of the h. pylori bacteria. I had spoken with Dr. Waltham after she had first seen Kathy; she, too, felt that Kathy's problem was gallbladder-related.

Kathy was obviously disappointed with the news that I had given her; one always hopes that there is a definitive answer for the suffering that you are experiencing, so that your physician can cure or manage the ailment producing your misery. However, I told her that I was still 100% convinced that she was trudging around with a "sick" gallbladder, and that, ultimately, she and that little bag of bile would need to part ways. That fact that the ultrasound had not demonstrated any stones did not deter me from my diagnosis. The bile that is manufactured by the liver differs in composition from person to person: so that the bile produced in one person may prove to be more irritating to the gallbladder lining than that manufactured in another individual. For Mr. Freeze, I ordered the nuclear medicine gallbladder scan for Thursday and a follow up on the following Monday. I carefully explained to her that, even if this subsequent test were to be "normal," I most likely would still recommend that she have Dr. Waltham perform a cholecystectomy (removal of the gallbladder), which she could do using a laparoscope. I explained that both she and I felt the same way about Kathy's problem based on her symptoms, our exam findings (which were classic for gallbladder inflammation), and the normal results of the other studies.

Kathy's nuclear medicine study was normal; we discussed her situation upon her return visit on Monday. I told her that, if she were my daughter, my wife, my grandmother, or even myself, I would recommend that she have a cholecystectomy performed. Her husband was with her at this visit; so that, for his benefit, I went through all of my reasoning again. Kathy finally said that she would call Dr. Waltham's office and schedule this surgery.

So now we ran into the "pigeonhole" problem with the insurance carrier. Kathy had not had "gallbladder colic," or an episode of acute cholecystitis, or pancreatitis leading to a hospitalization. In addition, all of her "gallbladder tests" were normal. Both Dr. Waltham and I had to submit all of our notes to the insurance carrier, and she had to talk with one of the more superior administrators before that person finally agreed to allow the surgery to go forward.

Dr. Waltham performed a laparoscopic cholecystectomy ten days later. At surgery she found that the gallbladder wall was greatly thickened. Kathy tolerated the surgery well and went home later that evening. The pathologist confirmed the presence of chronic gallbladder inflammation when he examined the specimen both grossly and under the microscope. Neither the surgeon nor the pathologist found stones in the organ, and all of the blood vessels were normal.

Three weeks passed before I next saw Kathy in the office. She had a big smile on her face when she told me that she now was having absolutely no gastrointestinal symptoms at all. Some patients develop diarrhea after their gallbladder has been removed; however, Kathy had escaped that complication. As I examined her abdomen once again, she simply smiled as I pressed into the previously tender area.

The "art" of medicine prevailed again in this case, in the face of normal scientific studies. It was this "art" that allowed us to snuff out the embers which had smoldered in this patient for a little over four months and had made her feel miserable. There was no "pigeonhole" here – just the physicians' careful attention to the patient's history and to their examination of the patient.

CHAPTER 17

"HAND ME MY WALKING STICK"

The above words are from a song by Leon Redbone, my favorite blues/jazz musician whom I followed for forty years until his retirement in March 2015, the same time that I retired. That brief snippet of the song's lyrics will serve to introduce my last topic. Unlike the other diseases, which were, for the most part, fairly rare, this problem is common – but often overlooked by the busy family physician. The embers of this disorder truly begin as barely a flicker, and stay that way for a number of years before it is possible for the physician to discern that they have begun to glow more brightly. For this problem is part of the aging process, which, as we all realize, develops over many years. As we age all of us gradually adapt to our "new normal," so that if we develop a new ache or pain, we reason that this is occurring because of our age.

For example, when I was young I could sit in the chair at this computer, raise my head up and see the ceiling. Now, with the arthritis in my neck, I can barely see the junction of the wall and the ceiling as I look up. That same neck arthritis is the reason that I now have to turn my entire body around if I wish to back up the car. If I get down on the floor in order to get my little dog's favorite toy out from under the TV stand, I then have to crawl over to a piece of furniture that will support me as I raise myself from the floor. I have a favorite 91-year-old woman that I cared for over a number of years; we were discussing this phenomenon during one of her visits, when she said, "Oh yes, Dr. Kassis; I call that 'furniture walking'."

As we age, we develop arthritis in multiple joints, including our neck, lower back, hips and knees, as well as in our hands – arthritis which is due to many years of use. The bones try to reinforce themselves by adding extra bone material; however, it is precisely this added bone that then produces pain and instability in the joints, as well as other problems if this extra bone is added to the vertebral joints. Because of the pain and instability in our hip and knee joints, our gait becomes somewhat unsteady, and we are prone to falls. The falls, however, are not just due to the arthritis in the joints; for, as we age, our reflexes – which were once brisk enough to allow us to catch ourselves, thereby preventing a fall – now are slowed to the point that, once we begin a fall, they no longer are able to stop the inevitable plunge downward.

In America there are approximately 200,000 hip fractures occurring in patients every year due to falls. Pelvic fractures also happen frequently as a result of such falls, which often seem to be relatively minor. (For example, I have suffered two pelvic fractures merely after tripping over my dog and falling onto the rug, fractures that gave me significant pain for six weeks before finally healing.) The patients with the hip fractures have it worse because they need surgery, with all of its potential perioperative complications, in order to regain their ambulatory ability – and many never do.

All of these disasters are likely to occur because the act of walking requires complex neurological functions: Our frontal lobes of the brain first have to decide where our feet are going to go, send that message down our spinal cord to the nerve cells in the lower back, which, in turn, initiate the movement of our legs in the desired direction. We also must maintain our balance, which is accomplished through a combination of our vision, input from the nerves in our feet, the balance mechanism of our inner ear, and the "coordination" part of our brain known as the cerebellum. In 2013 I received a medication that destroyed almost all of the balance mechanism of my inner ear; so that my brain no longer gets information from that region concerning my position in space, my head position, or if I AM in motion or not; I depend almost totally on my eyesight to furnish spatial information to my brain. The portion of my ear dedicated to hearing was not affected (although my wife, at times, would beg to differ.)   Because my brain lacks the input from my inner ear, I AM constantly off balance; at dusk or without the lights on I AM unable to walk, or even stand, without help. All day long I feel as if I AM trying to walk on an air mattress – a feeling of constant unsteadiness.   A patient with B12 deficiency develops degeneration in the nerves that tell their brain the position of their feet; so that he or she may have an ambulation problem similar to mine. Thus, one can see that, if any part of this mechanism is the least bit faulty, then our ability to maintain our balance while walking will suffer. When such a defect is combined with arthritis, we may lose our ability to walk altogether.

And so, every primary care physician will see at least four patients every day who are having trouble ambulating. Most of these patients will have one of the obvious reasons for the problem, e.g. bad hip or knee arthritis. But lurking among these patients is the one with the disorder that I mentioned above, and which is slowing progressing as the physician watches and assumes that one of the other problems is the reason for the walking disability. Once again, if the physician takes the history properly and does a decent neurological exam, then the diagnosis can be suspected and confirmed, leading to a referral and cure of the problem before that patient falls, sustains a fracture, and lands in a hospital where complications can easily arise.

Mary Sutton had been one of my patients for about nine years. She had hypertension, hypothyroidism, and mild arthritis of her knees, the latter giving her only minor discomfort. Since she had been doing well, I had not seen this 72- year-old, thin, active woman for about six months. Normally, she had no significant complaints; however, on the occasion of this visit she said, "Doc, I think that I'm developing a problem with my walking." As usual, I sat down on my stool and asked to her tell me about her symptoms.

"About eight months ago I began to feel like my feet just don't seem to want to go where I want them to. I didn't mention it at my last visit because I thought that it was merely due to my getting older. However, I feel that the problem has worsened over the last four months. I used to walk relatively fast for my age; but, as the last months have gone by, I find myself taking smaller steps and going more slowly. On one occasion the toe of my left foot caught the rug, and I fell; fortunately, I injured nothing but my pride. I AM not having any new aches or pains anywhere; but something is definitely wrong."

I questioned her about weight loss, fevers, night sweats, as well as about any symptoms referable to her heart, lungs, GI tract, and urinary systems; she had no problems with any of these. Now I aimed my questions toward her neurologic system. She reported no headaches, dizziness, or vision changes, nor had she noted any unilateral weakness of arm or leg. Although she had minor arthritic knees, Mary adamantly denied experiencing any neck pain, nor any pain radiating down either arm, nor pains radiating into her buttock region. Lastly, I asked if she having any numbness or tingling in her hands, legs, or feet; she answered "No." She had been taking her prescribed medications faithfully, and had not added any over-the-counter supplements.

Having completed my interrogation, I now began my exam. Since I would need to do a fairly detailed neurological examination, I saved that for the end and began the exam in my usual sequence.

Mary was a feisty woman who also had a great sense of humor. With blue eyes that sparkled and short grey hair, she only weighed 118 pounds. Her pulse, respirations and blood pressure were all normal – her blood pressure reading today was excellent at 122/68. My examination of her head, heart, lung and abdomen revealed no abnormalities; additionally, I found no enlarged lymph glands anywhere. Turning my attention to her extremities, I noted mild osteoarthritis in her hands and knees. Most importantly, I found that the range of motion of both hips was surprisingly normal for her age and that my manipulation of those joints caused her no pain.

So I now began the neurological exam. Mary's thinking ability was totally normal. Her eyes, ears, facial movements, and speech were also normal. I next tested her neck mobility, which I found to be extremely restricted by the arthritis that had developed over the years. She could barely raise her head up and could only turn her head about two inches toward each shoulder. As is usual in this condition, Mary could still flex her neck almost to the point that her chin closely approached her chest. Importantly, these maneuvers produced pain only when she extended her neck in order try to look at the ceiling, with the pain localizing to the back of the neck without radiation down the arms. (The picture below demonstrates the normal range of motion of the neck.) Next I tested the strength in her arms and legs along with her coordination, which were normal for her age; there was no tremor that might suggest Parkinson's disease.

So I now entered the last phase of the exam. I asked Mary to get off the exam table, go out into the hall, and walk to the end of the hall and then back into the exam room. I was now able to see her problem quite clearly; she walked with a very short, almost shuffling, stride. Her arm swings were normal – a fact which, once again – suggested that she did not have Parkinson's disease. She turned, walked back to the exam room, and climbed onto the exam table without assistance. I quickly tested her sensation to pain and vibration, both of which were normal.

Because I expected abnormalities, I saved my examination of her reflexes for the end of the evaluation. As you most likely know, your physician tests your reflexes by hitting certain muscle tendons of your body with the small hammer that is ever present in his or her lab coat. We actually grade the responses of your body to this assault with a score that ranges from 0 to 4+, with 0 being no response at all from the percussion to 4+, at which level the muscle twitches continuously for a number of seconds after having been struck only once by the hammer. When we are babies, all of our reflexes are 4+ because the brain has not yet firmly established all of its connections to the spinal cord in order to suppress these down to a normal level. At a level 2+ response (which we consider to be normal) the muscle will jerk once, and then relax again.

However, as we age, the nerve fibers going from the spinal cord to the muscles begin to degenerate; so that I would expect to find a 2+ reflex as I tested Mary's arm reflexes, while at her knees and ankles I would expect a response of 0 to 1+ at most. A significantly higher level obtained at the knees – and especially at the ankle site – would suggest that there is now a disconnect somewhere in the brain or spinal cord, resulting in the brain's inability to keep these local reflexes under control. If this is the case, then that disconnect may also allow the re-emergence of "primitive" reflexes, which were present prior to the brain's gaining mastery of the spinal cord; the finding of these types of reflexes in a patient confirms that a disconnect certainly is present, and their location often gives a clue as to where the problem lies.

I began testing Mary's reflexes in her arms, which were normal. Turning my attention to her lower extremities, I found a 3+ response both at the knees and the ankles – a level of response which I could obtain even by merely tapping the tendons with my finger. I now began my search for any "primitive" reflexes. These are reflexes that are present in all of us as infants. For example, if you startle a baby, the infant's arms will first extend and then come around toward the front of the infant as if the child were going to wrap its arms around something. This is not a purposeful act on the part of the infant; it is a reflex, the motions of which will occur in the same manner every time that infant is startled. As our brains mature and develop a more firm connection with the spinal cord nerves, the brain now becomes able to suppress these "primitive" reflexes, so that they are no longer discernable.

The first one of these that I sought is known as a "Babinski" response, in which scratching of the bottom of the foot causes the patient's big toe to rise while the other toes fan out. I found this test to be positive in both of Mary's feet. There is an analogous reflex that can be elicited in the hands, which, if present, localizes the problem to somewhere in the cervical spine – more precisely at levels 5-6. The "Hoffman reflex" is elicited by taking the middle finger of the hand and "flicking" the tip of the finger. If this reflex is present, the thumb will move toward the middle of the hand and the fingers will flex. The test was positive in Mary's left hand, but not in her right one; but, nevertheless, the combination of all of these findings now told me that Mary's ambulation difficulty was most likely due to pressure on her spinal cord in the neck produced by the very bad arthritis there – the presence of which I had already demonstrated by her exam. The spinal cord literally becomes squeezed by all of the extra bone that has developed in the neck joints over the years to the point where the brain is unable to get its commands via that compressed cord all the way down to the nerves that move the legs. The development of the neck arthritis is called "cervical spondylosis," while the compression of the spinal cord that it produces is known as "cervical myelopathy." It is this inability of the brain to now command the actions of the legs that leads to the gait problem, which develops very slowly in these patients – a gait disability that will ultimately cause a bad fall or even lead to their being wheel-chair-bound if the diagnosis is missed.

People who develop this condition often complain that their legs feel "stiff" when they walk, and that their feet just don't seem to want to go where they aim them. Because the disconnect in the neck area produces the stiffness (spasticity) in the legs, the toes are not lifted as with normal ambulation, so that the patient often finds that he or she trips over "nothing" -- hence the tendency to fall, with all of the potential complications arising from such an episode.

After I had finished Mary's examination, I brought in my anatomical model of a neck, which also demonstrated the spinal cord in that region. I carefully showed her the bony arch through which the spinal cord passed as well as the joints of the cervical vertebrae, which were now, with their arthritis, combining to narrow the diameter of that arch. The usual diameter of the arch (canal) at the level involved would measure at least 17-18 millimeters, while the spinal cord in this area is around 15 millimeters, the arch obviously being large enough for the cord to easily pass through. I told Mary that, based on my exam findings, I would expect to see her arch diameter on an MRI study to be in the range of 9-10 millimeters, with significant compression of her spinal cord because of that. I explained that I would need to do an MRI study of both her brain and of her cervical spine in order to be certain of the diagnosis. Lastly, I told her that, if I were correct in my diagnosis, I most likely would need to refer her to an excellent neurosurgeon who would be able to relieve this compression, thus allowing her to walk normally again. After all, she was a vibrant 72-year-old woman with no heart or lung problems; so I thought that she should be able to enjoy her life. "So this means that I'll have to have surgery on my neck?" she asked. "I have heard so many awful things about back surgery that I AM very much afraid of even considering that possibility." I attempted to reassure her; "What you have is a very common problem," I said. "Over my many years of practice I have seen at least one or two patients every month who have had the same problem as you do, and have referred hundreds of these people to a neurosurgeon for the surgery needed to open up the narrowed area. These patients have done well; so that I have no qualms about referring you if my diagnosis is proven to be correct." Without surgical intervention, the chances that she would be walking on her own in a year are slim. Patients often ask me what I would do if a family member or I were to have the same condition. My answer is always the same: "I treat all of my patients in the same manner that I would treat any of my family members or myself." If I were to have Mary's problem, I would call the neurosurgeon.

Mary finally agreed to have the further diagnostic studies done. I ordered lab work to check her blood count, conduct a complete chemistry profile, and provide a B12 level. Then I ordered an EKG to further look at her heart. I told Michelle to schedule Mary for an MRI of her brain with contrast, which was needed to rule out the presence of mini-strokes as well as a much rarer disease known as "Normal Pressure Hydrocephalus," both of which could affect her gait. Michelle also arranged for a non-contrast MRI of Mary's cervical spine, which would image the area in question. Since these would be completed over the next week, I arranged for Mary to follow up in ten days.

As is the case when one is busy, those ten days flew quickly by; I walked into my exam room to review all of the tests results with Mary and her daughter, who had accompanied her this time. I related that the results of all of the blood tests, including the B12 level, were normal and that she had an EKG of a 20-year-old woman. In addition, the MRI of her brain was that of a normal 72-year-old woman. I told her: "However, the MRI of your neck does not fall into the same wonderful category as do your other tests. It showed the narrowing that I suspected; but it proved to be even a bit worse than your exam suggested. The arch (canal) diameter is narrowed to a mere 9 millimeters both at the C4-5 and C5-6 levels." I reminded her, and now informed her daughter, that the normal canal diameter 17-18 millimeters. Thus, her 15 millimeter spinal cord is now being compressed by bone to a diameter of only 9 millimeters at the involved levels. As I looked at the MRI picture on the computer, the images were very striking indeed. As I stared at those pictures and reviewed her symptoms and my exam findings in my mind, I turned to Mary and her daughter and stated fairly firmly: "You need to have this area decompressed if you wish to continue walking. All of that extra bone which has formed over the years simply has to be removed in order to make room for the spinal cord. I have no medicine that can fix this, and no type of injection will make this problem go away."

The shock at being given this information was evident on both of their faces. Each looked at the other; finally, Dorothy, her daughter, asked, "What do you want to do, Mom?" Mary sat silently for a moment as she thought about this dilemma. Ultimately she looked at me and asked, "Do you have a surgeon whom you would recommend?" I responded by telling them that there were two excellent neurosurgeons, both in the same group in Abilene, to whom I send all of my patients needing neurosurgical expertise, and that I would be happy to get her an appointment with one of them. I reassured them that I had been very pleased over the years with their care of my patients, and that I would call either of them should I personally ever need their help. And so my staff made the referral, making certain that both Mary and her daughter knew to bring the MRI images with them to the appointment with Dr. Tad Talmage. I had already spoken with him and faxed all of my notes, along with her lab and X-ray reports, to his office.

I finally saw both Mary and her daughter back two months later. Her surgery had gone well, and she had to endure only a one-day stay in the hospital. Of course, the real question at this point that needed answering was, "How well are you able to walk now, Mary?" Her daughter broke in immediately. "Doc, she can outwalk me now." I turned to Mary and questioned her. "Is this true, Mary?" her smile was almost as broad as her face as she responded: "Doc, my legs are back to normal, and I can get around without any problem at all. Do you feel like racing?"

I briefly examined her; the "primitive" reflexes were now gone, although the hyperactive reflexes still persisted at her knees and ankles (given the severity of her cord compression, it would take about a year for these to return to normal). The remainder of her exam was stable. Mary did well even up to the time of my retirement. Fortunately for her, she never developed a similar problem in her lower back as so many of these patients go on to do. Thus another ember was discovered, and the disorder producing it treated effectively.

EPILOGUE

I hope that in this narrative I have given you, the reader, a glimpse into what the practice of medicine away from the bright lights and multiple subspecialists of the city has been like over my forty-year career. I also hope that I have exposed you to the fact that I was able to make the diagnosis of many of these smoldering illnesses by taking to heart the information provided by Mr. Sherlock Holmes and by Drs. Hamilton Bailey and Joseph Sapira. I also owe a great debt of gratitude to Dr. Hayden Ellingham not only for the unselfish sharing of his expertise with me during the early years of my practice, but also for his surgical skill in removing my Meckel's diverticulum, thus extinguishing my own ember that had burned for over 20 years. Lastly, I hope that I have shown you in this writing how special is the doctor-patient relationship. I worry that the current changes in medicine will forever alter that special bond by continuing to encroach upon the valuable time that physicians need to have with their patients – time which is sorely needed to obtain an accurate history, by which we are first able to potentially discern that which burns ever so slowly. However, this is just the "Geezer's" opinion.

Made in the USA
Coppell, TX
04 August 2020